Care of the Dying and Deceased Patient

The *Essential Clinical Skills for Nurses* series focuses on key clinical skills for nurses and other health professionals. These concise, accessible books assume no prior knowledge and focus on core clinical procedures and their rationale, together with the essential background theory. Their user-friendly format makes them an indispensable guide to clinical practice for all nurses, especially to student nurses and newly qualified staff.

Other titles in the *Essential Clinical Skills for Nurses* series:

Care of the Dying and Deceased Patient

A Practical Guide for Nurses

Edited by

Philip Jevon
RGN, BSc (Hons), PGCE, EB 124
Resuscitation Office/Clinical Skills Lead
Honorary Clinical Lecturer
Manor Hospital
Walsall
UK

WILEY-BLACKWELL
A John Wiley & Sons, Ltd., Publication

This edition first published 2010
© 2010 by Blackwell Publishing Ltd

Blackwell Publishing was acquired by John Wiley & Sons in February 2007.
Blackwell's publishing programme has been merged with Wiley's global
Scientific, Technical, and Medical business to form Wiley-Blackwell.

Registered office
John Wiley & Sons Ltd, The Atrium, Southern Gate, Chichester, West Sussex,
PO19 8SQ, United Kingdom

Editorial offices
9600 Garsington Road, Oxford, OX4 2DQ, United Kingdom
2121 State Avenue, Ames, Iowa 50014-8300, USA

For details of our global editorial offices, for customer services and for information about how to apply for permission to reuse the copyright material in
this book please see our website at www.wiley.com/wiley-blackwell.

Library of Congress Cataloging-in-Publication Data

Care of the dying and deceased patient / [edited by] Phil Jevon.
p. ; cm. – (Essential clinical skills for nurses)
Includes bibliographical references and index.
ISBN 978-1-4051-8339-0 (pbk. : alk. paper)
1. Terminal care. 2. Hospice nursing. I. Jevon, Philip. II. Series:
Essential clinical skills for nurses.
[DNLM: 1. Nursing Care–methods. 2. Terminal Care–methods.
3. Mortuary Practice. 4. Palliative Care–methods. 5. Patient Care
Planning. WY 152 C2713 2010]
RT87.T45C37 2010
616′.029–dc22
2009016399

A catalogue record for this book is available from the British Library.

Set in 9 on 11 pt Palatino by SNP Best-set Typesetter Ltd., Hong Kong
Printed and bound in Malaysia by KHL Printing Co Sdn Bhd

1 2010

Contents

Contents

Foreword

One of the most fulfilling yet challenging times in the career of a registered nurse is the moment they are faced with caring for a patient who is dying. This can be a daunting moment full of emotional tensions and anxieties, especially on the first occasion. However, it can be a fulfilling experience and it is a privilege to be able to care for a patient and their family during the latter stages of their lives. It is a challenge that utilises many skills in the nurse's toolbox, especially compassion and communication, to ensure a patient's final days are filled with privacy and dignity.

The care of the dying and the deceased patient is a complex situation as it requires skill to address the many emotional issues as well as complex clinical issues and legal requirements, especially around the issue of 'do not resuscitate'.

This book provides a comprehensive account of all of the areas that need to be considered and gives the registered nurse practical tips to deal with very emotive issues. It provides a holistic approach to care of the dying patient, encompassing a variety of areas from symptom control through to dealing with post mortems.

The book is easily navigated and its many contributors are to be congratulated on their work, which is evidence based and easy to comprehend.

It is with great pleasure that I recommend this book to you and I trust you will find it as interesting and informative as I did.

Brigid Stacey
Deputy Chief Executive/Chief Operation Officer/Nurse Director
Walsall Manor Hospital

Contributors

Liz Armstrong RGN, BSc (Hons)
West Midlands Regional Donor Transplant Coordinator, University Hospitals Birmingham NHS Trust

Fiona Foxall RGN, MA, BSc
Head of Continuing Education, University of Wolverhampton

Richard Griffith LLM BN PgdLaw DipN RMN CertEd,
Lecturer in Health Law, School of Health Science, Swansea University

Dan Higgins RGN, ENB 100, ENB 998
Senior Charge Nurse, Critical Care, Wellcome Building Critical Care, University Hospitals Birmingham NHS Foundation Trust; Consultant/Honorory Lecturer, Resuscitation Services UK Ltd; Visiting Clinical Lecturer, University of Birmingham

Rachel Hodge RGN
West Midlands Regional Donor Transplant Coordinator, University Hospitals Birmingham NHS Trust

Melanie Humphreys MA Research Methods, MA Medical Ethics and Law, BSc (Hons) Educational Studies (Nursing), ENB 124, DiPSiN, RGN, ONC
Director of Learning Beyond Registration & Blended Learning, Keele University

Louisa Hunwick RN, BSc in Specialist Practice/Health Visiting, Diploma in Counselling, ENB 998, ENB 937
Macmillan Palliative Care Nurse Specialist, Walsall Manor Hospital NHS Trust

Philip Jevon RGN, BSc (Hons), PGCE, ENB 124, DiPSiN
Resuscitation Officer/Clinical Skills Lead, Honorary Clinical Lecturer, Manor Hospital, Walsall

Shareen Juwle RN BSc (Hons)
Macmillan Palliative Care Nurse Specialist, Walsall Manor Hospital NHS Trust

Rachel McGuinness MIFPA BSc (Hons) Complementary Therapies
Lead Complementary Therapist for Palliative Care, NHS Walsall Community Health

Glen Mitchell RGN, BN (Hons) and ENB Higher Award,
Nurse Prescriber, Macmillan Palliative Care Nurse Specialist, Walsall Manor Hospital NHS Trust

Cassam Tengnah MSc, Post Graduate Diploma in Health Care Law, DN (London), Certificate in Education, RMN
Lecturer in Health Law, School of Health Science, Swansea University

Elaine Walton RGN, MSc, BSc (Hons), PGCE, ENB 124
Resuscitation Officer/Research Nurse Specialist, Manor Hospital, Walsall

Care of the Dying Patient: A Guide for Nurses

1

Dan Higgins

INTRODUCTION

Fifty-four per cent of deaths in England and Wales occur in acute hospital beds, 22% of people die at home and the remainder in other institutions, such as psychiatric hospitals (Office of National Statistics, 1999). Nearly 70% of deaths in the UK will be related to cancer, heart/circulatory disease and respiratory disease (Office of National Statistics, 2004). These figures imply that a significant proportion of patients will be receiving some form of care in the period prior to and at death, which necessitates health-care practitioners having the knowledge and skills to care for the dying patient. The pathway towards death may be a process of graduated illness involving many care services or completely unexpected, such as catastrophic trauma/cardiac arrest. The care needs of patients and their relatives, regardless of environment or cause or pathway, needs to be individualised and multifaceted to allow patients to approach death and to die free of symptoms and 'in peace' and to facilitate the support of bereft relatives.

The aim of this chapter is to provide an overview of the care of the dying patient.

LEARNING OUTCOMES

At the end of this chapter, the reader will be able to:

❏ Clearly define death and dying.
❏ Demonstrate an appreciation of the need for a multidisciplinary approach to care of the dying patient.
❏ Define and expand on nursing responsibilities and priorities in caring for the dying patient.
❏ Demonstrate an understanding of the Liverpool Care Pathway (LCP) for the dying patient and its implications for practice.

❏ Explore psychological, spiritual, social and religious/cultural aspects of care of the dying patient.
❏ Discuss the significance of and the treatment of symptom control in the care of the dying patient.
❏ Explore issues surrounding organ and tissue donation.
❏ Explore issues surrounding withdrawal of medical treatment.
❏ Discuss the role of palliative care nurse specialists.
❏ Discuss the role of support organisations in the care of the dying patient.
❏ Discuss the role of the hospice in the care of the dying patient.

DEFINING DEATH AND DYING

The current position in law is that there is no statutory definition of death in the UK (Department of Health (DH), 1998) owing to the fact that the definition of death is complex and subject to many influences.

One of the first documented definitions of death occurred as early as 1768 in the first edition of the *Encyclopaedia Britannica* (1973): 'Death is generally considered as the separation of the soul and body; in which sense it stands opposed to life, which consists in the union thereof'. Despite the phenomenal advances in science and technology since the 18th century, the earlier definition is the most approximate to how most lay individuals now conceptualise death.

Professional conceptualisation has been complicated. In early medicine, death was defined as the absence of respiratory sounds and an absence of heart sounds combined with unresponsiveness. However, these diagnostic criteria were easily challenged, firstly by certain recoverable conditions such as severe hypothermia/drowning and syncope mimicking death, and secondly by the development of cardiopulmonary resuscitation techniques. Descriptions of an individual 'returning to life' through 'resuscitation' were told in biblical times, and late 18th century scientific inquiry led to official reports of individuals being pronounced dead and being 'brought back to life'. Finally, moving into the 20th century, the development of artificial ventilators and cardiopulmonary bypass systems, and the use of pacemakers and organ transplantation became more commonplace; these developments confounded the definition of death further as patients could be kept 'alive' for periods of time.

The above-mentioned events led to the conceptualisation of death as a process rather than an assumption that the transformation from life to death was an instant one. In 1968, the Ad Hoc Committee of the Harvard Medical School (1968) defined brain death: 'A person is brain dead when he or she has suffered irreversible cessation of the functions of the entire brain, including the brain stem'. The report also outlined diagnostic criteria and the exclusion of preconditions for diagnosing brain death.

Determining death using neurological criteria, generally referred to as 'brain death', has been accepted for decades in most developed countries (Whetstine, 2007). However, the concept of equating brain death with 'death' has now been challenged, as brain dead individuals are at odds with our traditional intuition about death (Whetstine, 2007) and because of the physiological differences that exist between brain stem death and whole brain death.

The Department of Health (DH, 1998) recommended that the definition of death should be regarded as 'irreversible loss of the capacity for consciousness, combined with irreversible loss of the capacity to breathe'. The irreversible cessation of brain stem function produces this clinical state and therefore brain stem death equates with the death of the individual.

It is not inconceivable that advances in medical technology and knowledge may challenge this definition further in years to come.

Concept of a good death

Allowing a patient a 'good death' requires multidisciplinary, skilled and collaborative evidence-based care ranging from the simplest needs, such as positioning and communication, to advanced medical therapies.

The concept of a 'good death' is fluid and highly individual (Kehl, 2006). Bradbury (1999) suggests that a 'good death' can be described as a good 'sacred death', where one may die at peace 'spiritually', a good 'medicalised death', where there is freedom from pain and symptoms, or a good 'natural death', which is best conceptualised as passing away/passing on, or dying within sleep. However, these descriptions are not all-encompassing and may be subject to sociocultural variance and other influences. Kehl (2006), following a review of medical, nursing and patient perspectives as well as literature in sociology, suggests that individuals consider the following attributes as characteristic of a good death:

- Being in control.
- Being comfortable.
- A sense of closure.
- Trust in care providers.
- Recognition of impending death.
- Personal beliefs and values honoured.

A patient's perceptions of what he/she considers to be a good death must be explored to allow holistic care planning to meet his/her needs for a good death.

Principles of palliative care

The main priorities of nursing care in nursing the dying patient are to assist the individual to meet his or her personal needs leading up to death and to allow that individual a 'good' and 'peaceful' death.

The term 'palliative care', first proposed in 1974, encompasses this philosophy, moving the focus of care away from attempting to cure or preventing dying to improving the quality of life, through the prevention and relief of suffering in the time leading up to death. The World Health Organisation (www.who.int/en) suggests that palliative care:

- Provides relief from pain and other distressing symptoms.
- Affirms life and regards dying as a normal process.
- Intends neither to hasten nor postpone death.
- Integrates the psychological and spiritual aspects of patient care.
- Offers a support system to help patients live as actively as possible until death.
- Offers a support system to help the family cope during the patient's illness and in their own bereavement.
- Uses a team approach to address the needs of patients and their families, including bereavement counselling if indicated.

- Enhances quality of life and may also positively influence the course of illness.
- Is applicable early in the course of illness, in conjunction with other therapies that are intended to prolong life, such as chemotherapy or radiation therapy, and includes those investigations needed to better understand and manage distressing clinical complications.

A framework for meeting the fundamental nursing needs of the dying patient is suggested in Table 1.1.

Table 1.1 Key components of nursing care in nursing the dying patient

Core component/goal	Elements of care
Effective pain control	• Pain control is assessed continually • Administration of appropriate analgesia/analgesic delivery methods • Consideration of other methods of promoting comfort (heat pads/positioning, etc.) • Specialist advice is sought if necessary (e.g. a chronic pain service)
Patient is free from agitation/distress	• Continual assessment for agitation/distress • Providing an environment that allows the patient/family to communicate their fears/anxieties • Providing an environment that is conducive to privacy • Administration of appropriate anxiolytics as prescribed • Ensure that inappropriate interventions are discontinued
Patient is free from nausea/vomiting	• Continual assessment for nausea and vomiting • Administration of anti-emetic medication as appropriate/prescribed
Optimum management of any potential side effects of medication or management	• Appropriate nursing management of conditions such as dyspnoea, oedema and increased respiratory secretions • All nursing care to be delivered to reduce the risks of infection transmission
Optimum management of elimination/bowels	• Monitoring bowel movements • Enabling multidisciplinary management to avoid constipation/diarrhoea • Administration of appropriate medication as prescribed

Table 1.1 *Continued*

Core component/goal	Elements of care
Mobility/hygiene	• To avoid complications of immobility • Ongoing assessment of skin integrity • To prevent pressure ulcer formation • Utilisation of appropriate pressure relieving aids • Provision of hygiene needs, to include oral/eye care
Religious/spiritual needs	• Providing access to religious/spiritual support as required • The consideration of cultural needs in all aspects of care
Psychological support for the patient and his/her family	• The patient and his/her family are informed (as appropriate) of all procedures and care and the rationale for these • Assessment of the understanding of the patient's closest relatives, obtaining consent for passing on information • Ensure that patient and family are aware of treatment/care goals

MULTIDISCIPLINARY AND MULTI-AGENCY APPROACH IN CARING FOR THE DYING PATIENT

Multidisciplinary teams (MDT) are groups of professionals from similar and/or diverse disciplines who come together to provide comprehensive assessment, care and treatment for the patient. The team work collaboratively and cohesively to meet agreed objectives and outcomes. It would be difficult to argue that this approach is inferior to any other. However, it has been argued by Walton (2005) that health care in general is not routinely delivered by such teams and that the concept is more a theoretical ideal than a reality. At its best, the approach could meet the needs of patients and their relatives/significant others whilst developing staff and creating a process of ongoing improvement in the quality of care and clinical governance. However, if the MDT does not function effectively, care can become fragmented and outcomes could be detrimental to all concerned.

The size and composition of the MDT vary; complex cases such as those in palliative care may involve primary and secondary care teams, different agencies, including charitable organisations, and specialist palliative care services.

It is beyond the scope of this text to explore team structure and team dynamics; however, the basic fundamental component to any team approach to working is good multi-layered communication. Every MDT or service should implement processes to ensure effective inter-professional communication within teams, and between them and other service providers with whom the patient has contact (National Institute for Clinical Excellence (NICE), 2004).

Bliss *et al.* (2000) identified the key components to successful inter-professional working in palliative care as:

- Team members sharing a common medical and healthcare language.
- Individuals working within the team should be prepared to work together and not feel under threat from other professional groups.
- Individual team members placing value on the different contributions that can be made by each individual.
- A sharing of professional values and cultures.

Whilst these values are suggested for palliative care teams, they are essential for any team in order to meet the needs of any patient, not least in death.

The team should not be 'hospital-based', or 'community-based', but patient need-based. All MDTs and services should have mechanisms in place to gather the views of patients and carers on a regular basis (NICE, 2004), with every role and discipline being seen as an integral component. An overall team co-ordinator should be identified, although this individual must not be viewed as being 'the boss'; it should be an individual who communicates regularly with the patient and all members of the team. Mechanisms should be developed to promote continuity of care; this might include the nomination of a person to take on the role of 'key worker' for an individual patient (NICE, 2004).

The development of an MDT approach should be an ongoing process and should consist of collaborative meetings and training/education.

FRAMEWORKS FOR CARE OF THE DYING PATIENT

One of the key recommendations in the NICE document *Improving Supportive and Palliative Care for Adults with Cancer* (NICE, 2004) is that in all locations, the particular needs of patients who are dying from cancer should be identified and addressed. The Department of Health (DH, 2008) suggests the following three coordination processes for care of the dying patient.

Gold Standards Framework

The Gold Standards Framework (www.goldstandardsframework.nhs.uk) is designed to care for people with advanced, progressive, incurable illness, mainly in the primary care setting. It enables general practitioners (GPs) to identify patients for inclusion on the palliative care register. This approach helps primary care teams to work together in optimising continuity of care, teamwork, advance care planning, symptom control and patient, carer and staff support (DH, 2008).

Preferred Priorities for Care

The Preferred Priorities for Care (PPC) (www.endoflifecareforadults.nhs.uk) is a patient-held ambulatory document. It clearly outlines individuals' thoughts about their care and choices they would like to make. Preferred Priorities for Care aims to ensure seamless continuity of care, promote patient empowerment and provides the opportunity to discuss difficult issues that may not otherwise be addressed, to the detriment of patient care (DH, 2008).

Liverpool Care Pathway

The Liverpool Care Pathway (LCP) for the dying patient has been developed in the UK to transfer the hospice model of care of the dying into other care settings. It is a multiprofessional document that provides an evidence-based framework for care in the last days and hours of life, and is applicable to all care settings. The LCP is based on the principle of the integrated care pathway, a care method that aims to facilitate distinct care through integrated multidisciplinary cooperation (Veerbeek *et al.*, 2006). Integrated care pathways are structured care plans which detail essential steps in the care of patients with a specific clinical problem (Campbell *et al.*, 1998).

The pathway comprises three stages: initial assessment, ongoing assessment and after-death care. Each of these stages has specific evidence-based goals, which may or may not be achieved. If the goal is not achieved, it will be recorded as a variance from the normal plan of care. This, however, does not imply a failure in care; it may reflect care individualisation within the framework.

The LCP is designed for patients with life-limiting illness where the primary goal in care is provision of comfort. Multidisciplinary agreement should be made that if the patient is dying, all possible reversible causes for the current condition have been considered, and the patient may be two or more of the following:

- Bed-bound.
- Semi-conscious.
- Unable to take oral fluids.
- Unable to take tablets.

The key stages and patient goals of the LCP are demonstrated in Table 1.2.

Research evaluating the effectiveness of the LCP in practice is still relatively young, although promising. The pathway can facilitate 'simple' audit, for example which areas score highly in recorded variance, which can identify areas for future work, etc. Similar care pathways for the dying patient exist, such as the Supportive Care Pathway developed by the Pan Birmingham Palliative Care Network; again evaluation is in its infancy, although promising (Main *et al.*, 2006).

One of the key benefits of frameworks such as the LCP is that they are adaptable, in essence, to the clinical scenario, not least to cancer patients and those with long-term illness. The underlying principles of the programme should not be exclusive to cancer patients and should be considered for any patient meeting the above-mentioned criteria with life-limiting illness; this may include any end-stage organ system failure. Work is currently underway to explore the adaptability of the LCP to paediatrics, critical care, renal care and respiratory care scenarios.

Table 1.2 The Liverpool Care Pathway – Key stages and patient goals. Reproduced with kind permission of the Marie Curie Palliative Care Institute Liverpool (MCPCIL)

Stage	Focus/stage specifics	Assessment/patient goals
Initial assessment	Medical assessment, including the cessation of inappropriate therapy and medication, forward planning for treatment symptoms and an assessment of appropriate nursing care needs	• Physical assessment • Assessment of comfort • Psychological assessment • Assessment of psychological needs/insight into condition • Assessment of religious/spiritual needs • Assessment of communication needs
Ongoing assessment	Four-hourly nursing assessment of symptom control	• Pain • Agitation • Respiratory tract secretions • Nausea and emesis • Other symptoms such as dyspnoea • Oral hygiene • Elimination needs • Safe delivery of medication • Mobility/pressure area care • Psychological support • Religious/spiritual support • Needs of family/significant other
Care after death	Discussion with family Correct documentation	• Last offices • Property/valuables • Family information • Bereavement booklet • Informing GP/appropriate organisations

SYMPTOM CONTROL AND THE MANAGEMENT OF UNWANTED SIDE EFFECTS IN THE CARE OF THE DYING PATIENT

Disease processes and the management of a disease can produce a variety of symptoms and potential side effects. These symptoms may be physiological, psychological, social or spiritual in origin and may be influenced by many sociocultural variables. The effects of symptoms may be manifested in the dying patient who, by definition, may have little physiological reserve; this may result in severe distress. Many symptoms may be a result of medication and possible interactions between different medications. Multidisciplinary review of the patient's medication should occur throughout the dying phase to ensure that only drugs that are considered essential (those aimed at treating symptoms) should be administered. This may require the discontinuation of drugs previously considered essential, such as antihypertensives, etc.

When caring for the dying patient, the management of symptoms must be a high priority in order to improve the patient's and the family's experience of end-of-life care. Many cancer patient surveys demonstrate that symptom control has a high priority from both patients and carers (DH, 2000), and that the fear of inadequate control leads to severe distress (Steinhauser *et al.*, 2000).

It has been suggested that symptom assessment and control may be sub-optimal (NHS End of Life Care Programme, 2006) and differences may exist between primary and secondary care (Thomas, 2003), which may necessitate unwanted hospital admission. It has also been suggested that patients with organ system disease, such as chronic heart failure, miss out on the benefits provided to many cancer patients, particularly in relation to symptom control.

Cancer network-wide protocols and guidelines should be developed and implemented for symptom control (NICE, 2004), and these should be adaptable to other end-of-life disease situations. Certain tools have been devised for assessment of symptoms as part of the Gold Standards Framework and these are available from the website of the organisation (www. goldstandardsframework.nhs.uk). Many dying patients, particularly those in hospital, are not managed by the palliative care team and, as a result of this, the management of symptoms may not be optimal. An integrated care pathway provides one solution to this problem by giving the healthcare team a way to improve patients' access to high-quality symptom assessment and treatment in terminal care in general (Glare, 2003).

The diversity of symptoms that a patient may experience is particularly wide and specialist multidisciplinary advice should be sought from a variety of sources.

Symptoms that cause specific distress to patients include:

- Inadequate pain control.
- Agitation and distress.
- Increased respiratory tract secretions.
- Nausea and vomiting.
- Loss of appetite.
- Insomnia.
- Dyspnoea.
- Constipation.
- Urinary problems.

The first four in this list are the most common symptoms (Turner *et al.*, 1996) and these require specific mention.

Inadequate pain control

Individualised pain management in the dying patient should consist of: (a) identifying and treating the cause of pain if at all possible; (b) treating any factors that could be contributing toward pain, such as agitation and distress; (c) the use of appropriate analgesic agents, delivered via an appropriate route: and (d) the consideration of non-pharmacological pain relief.

The effectiveness of therapy should be evaluated at regular intervals, with the goal being pain control rather than pain relief.

Agitation and distress

Agitation, distress and delirium can compound other symptoms, particularly pain. Their presence can significantly reduce quality of life in the days/hours leading up to death. They may also cause distress to relatives and loved ones. Identifying and treating the cause of agitation is frequently difficult, particularly in the delirious patient or those with fluctuating levels of consciousness. Emotional distress is a predominant cause for distress and can be reduced by good communication and psychological support. Distress as a result of constipation/urinary retention or dyspnoea should be identified and treated accordingly. Metabolic disturbance, electrolyte/hydration imbalance and drug toxicity are also causes for altered mental state, although treatment may be more difficult. Glare (2003) suggests that correction of hypo/hyperglycaemia is the only metabolic derangement that is worth correcting in the last 48–72h of life. Pharmacological treatment for unresolved agitation and distress is common and this may consist of sedative and antipsychotic drugs.

Increased respiratory tract secretions
The phenomenon of noisy breathing in the hours before death is commonly referred to as the 'death rattle' and is a result of the movement of pooled respiratory secretions during respiration (Hugel *et al.*, 2006).

This may contribute to the development of terminal restlessness (Dickman, 2003). Treatment may consist of simple manoeuvres such as position change or suction; however, this may cause increased distress to the patient. The early introduction of antimuscarinic drugs may play a role in reducing secretions (Wildiers & Menten, 2002).

Nausea and vomiting
Many ill patients experience nausea, frequently without vomiting. It can occur in up to 62% of terminally ill patients with cancer (Rosseau, 2002). It may be exacerbated by gastro-intestinal problems, metabolic derangement or may be an adverse result of medication, particularly opiates. Although the causes are usually multifactorial, treatment should be aimed at any identified cause. Appropriate anti-emetic therapy should be initiated according to local drug guidelines.

The LCP recommends anticipatory medication prescribing for the top five symptoms that may be expected in the last hours/days of life. This enables a patient to receive medication appropriately without having to leave a patient in pain, for example whilst a doctor is contacted. Patient care and the management of symptoms may also improve with the advent of non-medical prescribing. (DH, 2006). Likewise, collaborative teamwork will be required to ensure that resources such as drugs, syringes and syringe drivers are available at the point of care.

PSYCHOLOGICAL, SOCIAL AND SPIRITUAL CARE OF THE DYING PATIENT

Psychological distress is common among people affected by cancer and is an understandable response to a traumatic and threatening experience (NICE, 2004). This distress often causes suffering in the patient nearing the end of life (Block, 2000). At the time of diagnosis of dying, approximately 50% of all patients experience anxiety and depression severe enough to affect their quality of life. In the subsequent 12 months, 1 in 10 people develop psychological symptoms severe enough to warrant specialist intervention (NICE, 2004). Although some literature discusses the psychological issues facing older patients and terminally ill patients with cancer, less is known about patients with end-stage pulmonary, cardiac, renal and neurologic disease (Block, 2000). The experiences of facing the end of life, regardless of disease process, are inevitably similar.

A large volume of work looking at patients' attitudes and responses towards death and dying or dealing with catastrophic news is influenced by the work of Elisabeth Kübler-Ross (1969), who suggested that patients journey, although not sequentially, within five stages of grief (as demonstrated in Box 1.1). This model has been criticised, not least because it considers all

---

Box 1.1 The five stages of grief according to Dr Elisabeth Kübler-Ross

- Denial: 'It can't be happening.' The initial stage of shock and numbness. A conscious or unconscious refusal to accept facts.
- Anger: 'Why me?' Anger may be internalised or externalised against the clinician, family or the individual's God.
- Bargaining: 'Just let me live to see my grandchild born.'
- Depression: The initial stages of acceptance.
- Acceptance: A stage where there may be some emotional detachment and objectivity.

These stages are not sequential and movement through the stages may be highly individualised and fluid

---

patients as experiencing similar pathways, and has limitations in its interpretation and development (Germain, 1980). However, the model does encompass a wide range of emotions that the dying patient, or bereft relatives, may experience. The psychological response to approaching the end of life will be influenced by a multitude of factors, including religion, faith, age, culture, social networks, finances and personal beliefs. To some, death may be welcomed, to others it may be feared.

Many patients utilise their family and social networks to express their views and fears. Some patients (the majority), however, are likely to benefit from additional professional intervention because of the level and nature of their distress (NICE, 2004). Providing psychological, social and spiritual care to the dying patient is a complex aspect of care provision, not least because these needs will be highly individualised. Care may also be influenced by the healthcare practitioner's knowledge, skills and attitudes regarding end-of-life care. Often, healthcare providers and families of dying patients are reluctant to accept that a dying individual's priority may be spiritual guidance, rather than technologically advanced medical care (Proulx & Jacelon, 2004). Trovo de Araujo & da Silva (2004) suggest that there are many different individual approaches in the endeavour to communicate with terminally ill patients, including avoidance patterns, which may be a result of personal difficulties in coping with the reality of human suffering and death.

The underlying principle in providing psychological, social and spiritual care to the dying patient is good communication, which leads to dynamic assessment and planning of end-of-life care.

Psychological care

Providing psychological support to help patients to face death should begin at the point of diagnosis; to a large proportion of patients this may be a time of severe shock and disbelief that 'this is happening to them'. They may have many questions that need answering honestly. Assessing psychological needs should begin with assessing patients' insights into their condition. Many patients who have been informed that 'they are going to die as a result of the illness' may have little knowledge of this fact.

Information provided may have been delivered badly, misinterpreted or misheard from initial discussion. Assessing insight informs the practitioner what information/services may be required. Issues related to dying and death should be explored appropriately and sensitively. Callanan & Kelley (1992) insist on the value of honesty in the nurse–patient relationship when describing the physiological process the patient experiences.

NICE (2004) recommend a four-level model of psychological assessment and intervention (Table 1.3). In this model, the patient progresses through four stages of assessment/care, starting with healthcare professionals at all levels, progressing to mental health specialists. The model may have many advantages, not least in providing access to highly trained practitioners with considera-

Table 1.3 The four-level model of psychological assessment and intervention

Level	Group	Assessment	Intervention
1	All health and social care professionals	Recognising psychological needs	Effective information giving, compassionate communication and general psychological support
2	Health- and social care professionals with additional expertise	Screening for psychological distress	Psychological techniques such as problem-solving
3	Trained and accredited professionals	Assessing psychological distress and diagnosis of some psychopathology	Counselling and specific psychological interventions such as anxiety and solution-focused therapy, delivered according to a specific theoretical framework
4	Mental health specialists	Diagnosis of psychopathology	Specialist psychological and psychiatric interventions such as psychotherapy and cognitive behavioural therapy

ble experience in psychological assessment and care. It also allows for patient needs to be met by a variety of sources. However, unless good communication exists between the professional groups, the model is futile, as care will fragment.

Price *et al.* (2006) suggest that delivery of the NICE guidelines, regarding the provision of psychological support, may be compromised by limited availability of specialist services and that this area needs further research.

Social care

As individuals approach the end of life, they may draw on the support of their family, friends and loved ones or 'significant others'. Healthcare practitioners have a responsibility to provide support for these individuals and be aware that family members will also be progressing through stages of grief and impending loss and will have their own psychological needs. The family's insight into the patient's condition should be assessed, and issues relating to dying and death explored appropriately and sensitively (Ellershaw & Ward, 2003). However, staff must be aware of breaching confidentiality and ensure that information is provided with a person's consent if he/she is able to provide it. Healthcare staff must ensure that ambiguous language is avoided when communicating with relatives. Relatives should be aware that the patient is going to die and that treatment and care is directed at allowing a good death. Questions should be encouraged and opportunities given for them to spend time with the patient. Relatives should be able to access support in the time leading up to death and following death. To provide a broader aspect of social care, communication should exist between the MDT and social care organisations, whose services impact on patient well-being both during the time leading up to and after death. This may include advice regarding financial arrangements and continuing care services.

Spiritual and religious care

Spirituality can be defined as, 'a search for existential meaning within a life experience, usually with reference to a power other than self, not necessarily called "God", which enables transcendence and hope' (Ellershaw & Wilkinson, 2003).

Religion can be defined as, 'belief in, worship and faith in a supernatural power which controls human destiny.'

Evidence suggests that religious and spiritual issues are significant for many patients and their carers in the last year of their life and that most patients' spiritual needs centre around their loss of role, self-identity and their fear of dying (Murray *et al.*, 2004). The needs of patients for spiritual support are, however, frequently unrecognised by health and social care professionals, who might feel uncomfortable broaching spiritual issues (NICE, 2004).

Providing spiritual care cannot be undertaken by only determining the patient's religion. A person's spirituality may or may not be religious in its foundation; a non-religious person may still have deep spirituality and spiritual needs (Speck *et al.*, 2004). To meet a patient's religious and spiritual needs, a comprehensive assessment is required, and this process needs to be continually reassessed throughout care as needs differ and change throughout the process leading up to death.

Healthcare staff need to be sensitive to, and have an awareness of, many cultural and religious backgrounds to better facilitate care. Staff also need to be able to value individuals' relationships with their chosen faith, beliefs and values. Healthcare staff have a responsibility to provide access to qualified, authorised and appointed spiritual care. They should also be aware of local community resources for spiritual care (NICE, 2004).

Formal religious traditions may have to be observed in the dying phase and may also influence care of the body after death (Ellershaw & Ward, 2003). Observing these traditions may also play an important role in the relatives' grieving process and acceptance of death.

Certain cultural and religious groups view death in different ways and employ certain practices with regard to death, dying and bereavement. A brief overview of some of these practices/views is presented in Table 1.4. However, these will be subject to various influences and should not be treated as definitive.

WITHDRAWAL OF MEDICAL TREATMENT
In any medical setting, the most important factors that must be considered in determining a treatment plan are the wishes and

Table 1.4 Some religious/cultural considerations when caring for the dying patient. Adapted from *Death with Dignity* (Green, 1993)

Religion	Common themes
Islamic (Muslim)	• Approaching death, close friends and family spend time in attendance to help the dying person to iterate his or her commitment to unity of God via prayer. This group may be large in comparison, with traditional views of 'close family and friends' • The dying patient may wish to lie with his or her face towards Mecca (the religious centre for Muslims) • Sick patients are not expected to fast during the month of Ramadan • Muslim relatives may request that the body is not touched by non-Muslim hands and therefore gloves should be worn during last offices • On death, the body is washed and wrapped in a shroud. Muslims gather and a prayer is performed for the dead • The body is buried (not cremated), with the head facing Mecca, as soon as possible • Charity, fasting, prayers and pilgrimage are often performed on behalf of the dead • Some confusion exists around organ donation as this interferes with burying the body as soon as possible • Post mortems are likewise not welcomed • If referring to the Coroner, identify religion as this may allow more prompt release of the body
Hinduism	• During end of life, devout Hindus may receive some comfort from readings from the Hindu holy texts • A Hindu priest may scatter holy water, tie a thread around the wrist or place a sacred leaf on the person • Hindu relatives may request that the body is not touched by non-Hindu hands and therefore gloves should be worn during last offices • Jewellry/threads should not be removed • After death, cremation is usual for adults, although children may be buried • Many Hindus prefer to die at home • Close relatives of the deceased may observe a 13-day mourning period.Close relatives may wish to spread the deceased person's ashes in the River Ganges. • Close male relatives of the deceased may shave their heads as a mark of respect. • Cremation should occur as soon as possible. • No objection is generally expressed towards organ donation/post mortem, although the latter is disliked

Table 1.4 *Continued*

Religion	Common themes
Judiasm	• A dying Jew may wish to hear psalms being sung or a special prayer (The Shema). They may also wish to hold the page of the Psalm or prayer. • At death, the child of the deceased may wish to close the eyes, this should be done as soon as possible after death. • Burial should occur within 24 h although not during the Sabbath (nightfall on Friday until Saturday evening). Some more liberal Jews wish to be cremated. • If death occurs during the Sabbath, many orthodox Jews may resent moving the body until it is over. • If a Coroner's referral is necessary, he should be informed about the body • Following death, immediate family may stay and mourn at home for 7 days. • Generally, no objection is expressed towards organ donation although this may differ in orthodox Jews.
Sikhism	• During the end of life, some Sikhs may receive comfort from readings from Guru Granth Sahib (The Sikh Holy book) • After death, many Sikh families may wish to attend to last offices themselves. • During last offices, the hair should not remain covered (under no circumstances cut). • Sikhs are usually cremated and have a preference for this to take place as soon as possible after death. Small children and babies may be buried • No objection is generally expressed towards organ donation
Buddism	• The important consideration is the state of the mind prior to death, which ideally will be a time of peace. Drugs which sedate or cloud conscious level may be refused. • At the time of death, it is important to inform a Buddist monk or a Minister as soon as possible. • Most Buddists prefer cremation. • No objection is generally expressed towards organ donation/transplantation or post mortem.

autonomy of the patient (Kinoshita, 2007). Underlying this principle is the issue of informed consent. Information should be provided to the patient, including benefits/negative effects, probability of effectiveness and potential alternatives to a treatment in order for the patient to make a balanced decision regarding whether the treatment is wanted or not. The MDT has a responsibility to ascertain that the patient is competent to make that decision, according to guidelines outlined in the Mental Capacity Act (Department for Constitutional Affairs, 2005). Patients may wish to change their minds about the treatment once it has begun and therefore should be provided with all the necessary information and their wishes adhered to.

Many patients are competent to express their views and issue directives regarding their medical care and treatment, particularly those in progressive disease processes. However, many patients die as a result of a catastrophic, short-term illness, necessitating 'artificial life support' therapy and are not able to make these decisions. Likewise, patients may become unconscious as result of treatment/disease and cannot make their own decisions. In this case, the Mental Capacity Act should be consulted. (The basic principles of the Mental Capacity Act are demonstrated in Box 1.2.)

Box 1.2 The Mental Capacity Act (2007)

The main changes as a result of the act are:

- There will be a single clear test for assessing whether a person lacks capacity to make a decision.
- The provision of ways in which individuals can influence what happens to them in the future, such as Lasting Power of Attorney (LPA), advance decisions, etc. An LPA will allow people over the age of 18 to formally appoint someone to look after their health, welfare and/or financial decisions.
- The clarification of what actions need to be taken when someone lacks capacity.
- Obligation to consult everyone involved in someone's care/ interested in their welfare.

The central components of the act are:

- Every adult has the right to make their own decisions and be assumed to have capacity to do so unless proved otherwise.
- People must be supported as much as possible to make their own decisions before anyone concludes they cannot do so.

Continued

- People have the right to make what others might regard as unwise or eccentric decisions.
- Anything done for, or on behalf of, people who lack mental capacity must be done in their best interests.
- Anything done for, or on behalf of, people without capacity should be the least restrictive of their basic rights and freedoms.

With regard to acting in a patient's best interests, the decision-maker should:

- Not make assumptions about someone's best interests based merely on age, appearance or behaviour.
- Consider all the relevant circumstances relating to the decision in question.
- Consider if a person is likely to regain capacity – can the decision wait until then?
- Involve the person as fully as possible in the decision that is being made on his or her behalf.
- With regard to withdrawal of life-sustaining treatment, the decision-maker must not be motivated by a desire to bring about the person's death.

Patient decisions regarding refusal of treatment must be:

- Valid.
- Applicable to the treatment in question.
- In writing.
- Signed and witnessed.

A patient cannot:

- Make an advance decision to ask for medical treatment.
- Make an advance decision to ask for their life to be ended.

This also applies to the initiation of cardiopulmonary resuscitation in the event of cardiac arrest. Current medical emphasis on autonomy requires that patients be primary in authorising do-not-resuscitate orders (Elliot & Olver, 2007), yet this may not always be achievable.

Any medical treatment must follow the ethical principles of beneficence and non-maleficence (Eschun *et al.*, 1999). In many cases, it can be argued that the continuation of medical treatment and intervention is not in the best interests of the patient. This is particularly relevant in patients approaching the end of life through disease and ill health, most notably organ system failure and cancer. Thus the most appropriate route of care may be the withdrawal of treatment.

Withdrawal of treatment is not uncommon in certain clinical settings, yet little work has been published exploring the issue that is, in the main, applicable to intensive care scenarios. There are numerous ethical and legal dilemmas associated with withdrawal of treatment, as was demonstrated in the Tony Bland case of the early 1990s where the question what constitutes medical treatment was raised (Howe, 2006). Withdrawal of treatment can vary from the discontinuation of antibiotics to the withdrawal of advanced renal/cardiovascular support. What should not be withdrawn is analgesia and treatment aimed at reducing distress and any symptoms.

The most important component of withdrawal of treatment is that it does not equate with withdrawal of care. Care to ensure the comfort of a dying patient is as important as the preceding attempts to achieve cure (Winter & Cohen, 1999).

The following criteria should be present when considering the withdrawal of treatment:

A situation where continued treatment would provide no overall benefit to the patient and may prolong unnecessary suffering.

or

A situation where there is irrefutable evidence that brain stem death has occurred.

The overall responsibility for withdrawal of treatment is with the patient's consultant. However, multidisciplinary discussion and agreement should be sought. In the UK, the patient's relatives do not have legal rights of decision-making (Winter & Cohen, 1999), but this should not exclude them from these discussions. It is imperative that relatives comprehend that they do not have to make a decision as this may be perceived as an overwhelming burden placed on them.

In accordance with the Mental Capacity Act, a Lasting Power of Attorney (LPA) has the right to make decisions regarding the initiation of life-saving treatment (such as cardiopulmonary resuscitation) and the withdrawal of life-sustaining treatment, only if this is specified in the legal documentation. An LPA may wish to continue medical treatment despite discordance with what is perceived as in the patient's best interests. The final responsibility for deciding what is in a person's best interest lies with the member of healthcare staff responsible for the person's treatment (the consultant). If agreement cannot be reached through excellence in communication, an application may be made to the court of protection.

Difficulties may arise in the withdrawal of treatment if:

(1) The patient requests discontinuation of therapy.
(2) The patient's family requests continued futile therapy.
(3) There is a lack of multidisciplinary agreement about withdrawal.

Appropriate communication with regard to the rationale of decision-making must be fully explained to relatives, with particular emphasis on the duty of care to the patient and the patient's best interests.

The MDT may often have differences of opinion with regard to withdrawal; again 'what is in the patient's best interest' should be the essential component of any discussions. Senior clinical experts should be involved in all discussions.

ORGAN DONATION

The role of organ and tissue transplantation in health care is well established and continues to develop as a result of advances in technology, surgical technique and immunosuppressant therapy. Currently, the demand for transplant organs, particularly kidneys, far exceeds the supply in the UK (Darr & Randhawa, 1999). The number of transplants performed in the UK has remained virtually static over the last 10 years; during this interval, the number of donors has decreased by approximately 20% (DH, 2004).

The supply of organs for donation usually comes from three sources:

• A 'heart beating' donor that is certified as brain stem dead on respiratory support.

- A living person who consents to organ donation.
- A non-heart beating donor.

The brain stem dead patient

Damage to the brain stem may occur as a result of intracranial or extracranial insult, the common causes being intracranial hypertension, trauma and cerebral anoxia. In many unconscious, unresponsive patients cardiopulmonary support is initiated and brain stem dysfunction realised after the event. In these patients, brain stem testing in line with the code of practice for the diagnosis of brain stem death (DH, 1998) is appropriate.

According to this code of practice, a patient may be certified as brain stem dead when:

- There is no doubt that the patient's condition is due to irremediable brain damage of known aetiology.
- The patient is deeply unconscious.
- There is no evidence that the state is due to depressant drugs.
- Primary hypothermia as the cause of unconsciousness has been excluded.
- Potentially reversible circulatory, metabolic and endocrine disturbances have been excluded as the cause of the continuation of unconsciousness.
- The patient is being maintained on the ventilator because spontaneous respiration has been inadequate or ceased altogether.
- All brain stem reflexes are absent.

When brain stem death has been established by the methods outlined in the code of practice, the patient is dead even though respiration and circulation can be artificially maintained (DH, 1998). At this stage, it becomes appropriate to consider whether any of the dead patient's organs can be made available for transplant prior to discontinuation of cardiopulmonary support (DH, 1998). If organ donation is not appropriate, cardiopulmonary support is discontinued at the completion of a second set of brain stem death tests. For legal purposes, the time of death is recorded as the completion of the first set of tests.

It is pertinent to emphasise that whilst cardiac and circulatory function may continue in the brain dead patient, the pathophysiological processes associated with brain stem death result in cessation of heart beat over a short period of time.

Obviously, consent for organ donation cannot be expressed by the patient. Consent may be assumed if a patient has expressed a wish to donate organs prior to illness; the generally accepted route of doing so is via the organ donor register or by carrying a donor card, although many individuals express wishes to their close family. In a case of a person who has signed the organ donor register, family members have no legal right to veto this person's wishes (Human Tissue Act, 2004), although this situation requires exceptionally skilled handling and communication from a healthcare team. If a patient has been certified as brain stem dead on the first set of tests, it is usual practice for the family to be approached by healthcare staff to explore what the patient's views were towards organ donation; again this process requires exceptional communication skills. Most transplant centres employ procurement transplant co-ordinators who have immense experience and skills in this field and they should be consulted at the earliest opportunity.

Brain stem death and the process of organ donation from a brain stem dead patient is particularly traumatic for relatives, as their perceptions of how their relative appears on the intensive care unit differs from their preconceived perceptions of a 'dead person'. Again, excellent communication and possible in-depth discussion regarding perceptions of death need to be ventured into.

Non-heart beating donation

Organ transplantation originated in taking organs from people who had recently died, but many of these transplants failed because organs had suffered damage as a result of ischaemia. Necessitated by the increasing demand for organs, organ retrieval shortly following the moment of cardiorespiratory death (non-heart beating organ donation) is now being revisited. The advantage of the system is that the patient is able to provide consent for organ donation or can make an advanced directive to this effect.

Although the re-visitation of this process is in its infancy, the process typically occurs in critical care units where active treatment has been withdrawn. When this occurs, a transplant co-ordinator is contacted and suitability for non-heart beating organ or tissue donation is assessed. Death is certified following loss of cardiorespiratory function. The body is cooled aggressively and taken to theatre for organ retrieval. In some cases, femoral arteries are cannulated prior to death, which reduces ischaemic time. The process is predominantly used for kidney donation.

However, there are many implications and concerns with non-heart beating donation. First and foremost is the concept of death as a process and the differences between cardiopulmonary death and neurological death. It could be questioned whether death has really occurred. This is complicated further by a situation known as the Lazarus effect, where some cardiac function returns some time after asystole and the withdrawal of resuscitative measures (Maleck *et al.*, 1998; Adhiyaman & Sundaram, 2007). It is accepted by the British Transplant Society that an interval of five minutes between the cessation of cardiopulmonary function and the declaration of death provides adequate assurance of the irreversible cessation of cardiopulmonary function (British Transplant Society, 2004).

Other considerations are practical and cost-based, with regard to place of care and withdrawal of treatment, intensive care resources and theatre time and availability. Whilst questions about non-heart beating donation exist, there has been a 20% increase in non-heart beating organ donation in recent years (DH, 2004).

Living donation

Living donation, whilst not directly related to care of the dying patient, should be mentioned. This occurs when an individual consents to removal of a healthy organ to a person of the same tissue type as themselves. The donor is usually a relative, and the practice is predominant in kidney transplantation, although tissue such as bone marrow can be transplanted. The practice has extended to individuals donating organs to people they do not know and has even occurred via the internet (Olsen, 2007), although to donate an organ for financial gain is illegal in the UK.

THE ROLE OF PALLIATIVE SPECIALISTS IN CARING FOR THE DYING PATIENT

Specialist palliative care services, largely funded by the voluntary sector, have enhanced the quality of care given to dying patients throughout the world and improved our level of knowledge and understanding of the art and science of palliative care (Thomas, 2003). There may still be room for improvement, as those with 'non-cancer' end stage diagnoses such as heart failure, chronic obstructive pulmonary disease, renal failure, neurological disease and dementia, who have equally severe symptoms with similarly poor prognoses, may have reduced access to services or specialist advice (Thomas, 2003). There is also acknowledgement that support for patients living at home with advanced cancer is sometimes poorly coordinated and may not be available over 24 h (Storey *et al.*, 2003). Whilst not denying the substantial role that these organisations play in palliative care delivery in all settings, it could be suggested that a reliance on voluntary funding could be a contributing factor hindering improvements in care. There is also a need for hospital and community-based MDTs to embrace the clinical expertise and experiences of some of these services.

To list and describe organisations that have input into palliative care would be overwhelming and beyond the scope of this text. The role of two prominent organisations in cancer care is described further.

Macmillan Cancer Support

Macmillan Cancer Support is a voluntary-funded organisation founded originally as The Society for the Prevention and Relief of Cancer by Douglas Macmillan in 1911 as a response to him witnessing his father's pain and suffering as a result of cancer. Since its formation, the organisation has contributed significantly to developments in cancer care, making contributions to building hospices, funding nursing and medical posts, and providing multidisciplinary training and education. In 2005, the number of Macmillan multidisciplinary health professionals rose to 3500. The organisation is multifaceted and provides social, emotional, financial and practical support for those with cancer. The involvement of Macmillan professionals should begin at the diagnosis of cancer and can continue up until death, with continuing support for bereaved families after death.

Marie Curie Cancer Care

Marie Curie Cancer Care was established in 1948 and is now one of the UK's largest health charities. It employs nearly 3000 healthcare professionals and provides free direct and indirect care to around 25000 people with cancer annually. The organisation does not focus solely on cancer and helps individuals nearing the end of life through other organ system failure/disease processes. There are three main inter-linking aspects of work: (1) nursing, (2) Marie Curie hospices and (3) research into both cancer and palliative care.

One of the aims of Marie Curie Cancer Care is to allow patients requiring end-of-life care to die at home if this is their wish. Sixty-five per cent of people with cancer want to die at home; at present only about 30% are successful in doing so (Higginson & Sen-Gupta, 2000) This may be because the place of final care for patients with terminal illness is influenced more by resource availability than patient choice (Storey *et al.*, 2003). Marie Curie nurses deliver direct care to patients, providing respite for carers, often overnight. This may often negate the need for hospital admission.

Marie Curie Cancer Care has 10 hospices throughout the UK, offering day therapy, complementary therapies and specialist care.

Other palliative care specialists

There are many individuals who contribute to palliative care both generally and within specific disease frameworks. This includes oncologists, pain specialists and nurses specialising in fields such as upper gastro-intestinal disease, breast care and stoma care. The role of these individuals cannot be understated.

SUPPORT ORGANISATIONS

There are many support organisations that may play a large role in caring for the dying patient; services offered by these organisations can be wide ranging, from direct care provision and advice to providing somebody to talk to.

Some hospice organisations offer a bereavement follow-up service for bereft relatives. Access to the majority of these organisations is usually free and increasingly easy through the internet.

Table 1.5 is a list of some useful organisations and general contact advice; the list is by no means exclusive and any omission is unintentional.

ROLE OF THE HOSPICE IN THE CARE OF THE DYING PATIENT

The concept of hospice care was developed as a reaction against the medical model of disease, diagnosis and cure (Clarke, 2002). Integral to this development process was Dame Cicely Saunders, who has been credited with founding the hospice movement and playing a key role in revolutionising care of the dying in the UK. The first hospice, St Christopher's Hospice in London, opened in

Table 1.5 Support organisations

Organisation	Service provided	Contact
Cancerbackup	Europe's leading cancer information charity, with over 6500 pages of up-to-date cancer information, practical advice and support for cancer patients, their families and carers	www.cancerbackup.org.uk 0808 800 1234
Marie Curie Cancer Care	Marie Curie nurses provide free nursing care to cancer patients and those with other terminal illnesses in their own homes	www.mariecurie.org.uk 0800 716 146.
Macmillan Cancer Support	Practical, medical, emotional and financial support	www.macmillan.org.uk CancerLine 0808 808 2020 Macmillan YouthLine 0808 808 0800

Table 1.5 *Continued*

Organisation	Service provided	Contact
The Samaritans	Confidential, emotional support, 24 h a day for people who are experiencing feelings of distress or despair, including those which could lead to suicide	www.samaritans.org.uk 0845 790 9090
NHS Direct	Telephone and e-health information services day and night direct to the public	www.nhsdirect.nhs.uk 0845 4647
ACT (Association for Children with Life-threatening or Terminal Conditions and their Families)	Information on support services for families whose children have life-threatening or terminal conditions	www.act.org.uk Information line 0117 922 1556
Breast Cancer Care	Support and information for women with breast cancer or other breast-related problems	www.breastcancercare.org.uk Helpline 0808 800 6000
British Red Cross Society	Local services including transport and escort, medical loan and domiciliary care	www.redcross.org.uk 020 7235 5454
Cruse Bereavement Care	Help to people bereaved by death. Free counselling service. Opportunities for contact with others through bereavement support groups and advice	www.crusebereavementcare.org.uk
Hospice Information	Publishes a directory of hospice and palliative care services	www.hospiceinformation.info 0870 903 3903
Sue Ryder Care	Services include long-term care, respite care, symptom control, rehabilitation, day care and domiciliary care	www.suerydercare.org 020 7400 0440

1967. This hospice, and its approach to end-of-life care, became an inspiration to other healthcare areas (Clarke, 2002) and the hospice model of care has grown into a worldwide movement that has greatly influenced care for those with end-stage diseases and cancer, and those requiring end-of-life care. The general philosophy of hospice care is the affirmation of death as a natural part of life, and holistic care is delivered meeting physical, emotional, social and spiritual needs as patients approach the end of life. Hospices are staffed by MDTs, who strive to offer freedom from pain and symptoms as a result of disease, and to provide dignity and peace at the end of life.

There is a general impression that a hospice is a place where people go to die. Evidence refutes this: approximately 50% of patients admitted to a hospice are discharged, the majority of whom are discharged home (National Council for Palliative Care, 2006). This may be because aspects of care, such as symptom control, are specific; sometimes complementary therapies can be offered by hospices and patients may be admitted for these reasons. Respite care and day care is also frequently available.

All hospice care is free of charge, yet many organisations rely upon fundraising and charitable donations to maintain high standards. The hospice philosophy and models of care are adaptable for use in the community and hospital setting; modification of hospice models such as the LCP is one approach to improve palliative care in all settings. The hospice approach to care has also led to ventures such as the hospice at home (National Forum for Hospice at Home, UK, www.hospiceathome.org.uk/), allowing patients to die at home with a comprehensive hospice-based care package. Today the word 'hospice' is synonymous with quality care towards the end of life; the challenge is to transfer that synonymity into all healthcare settings.

CONCLUSION

Meeting the care needs of the dying patient is complex and highly individualised. It is influenced by social, cultural, religious and spiritual factors. Other influences include legal, moral and ethical issues, and the attitudes of care givers themselves.

Maintaining high standards in caring for the dying patient is the responsibility of all the MDT and each individual member working towards a shared goal of allowing a good death as perceived by that patient and supporting his or her bereft relatives.

Excellent, multilayered communication through all mediums is the key skill required to meet these responsibilities.

REFERENCES

Ad Hoc Committee of the Harvard Medical School to Examine the Definition of Brain Death (1968) A definition of irreversible coma. *JAMA* **205**: 337–340.

Adhiyaman V, Sundaram R (2007) The Lazarus phenomenon. *J R Coll Physicians Ed* **32**: 9–13.

Bliss J, Cowley S, While A (2000) Interprofessional working in palliative care in the community: A review of the literature. *J Interprofess Care* **14**(3): 281–290.

Block SD (2000) Assessing and managing depression in the terminally ill patient. *Ann Intern Med* **132**: 3.y.

Bradbury M (1999) *Representations of Death: A Social Psychological Perspective*. Routledge, New York.

British Transplant Society (2004) *Guidelines Relating to Solid Organ Transplants from Non-Heart Beating Donors*. British Transplant Society, London.

Callanan M, Kelley P (1992) *Final Gifts: Understanding the Special Awareness, Needs, and Communications of the Dying*. Poseidon Press, New York.

Campbell H, Hotchkiss R, Bradshaw N, Porteous M (1998) Integrated care pathways. *BMJ* **316**: 133–137.

Clarke D (2002) Between hope and acceptance: The medicalisation of dying. *BMJ* **324**: 905–907.

Darr A, Randhawa G (1999) Awareness and attitudes towards organ donation and transplantation among the Asian population: A preliminary survey in Luton, UK. *Transplant Int* **12**: 365–371.

Department for Constitutional Affairs (2005) *The Mental Capacity Act: Code of Practice*. The Stationary Office, London.

Department of Health (DH) (1998) *A Code of Practice for the Diagnosis of Brain Stem Death including the Guidelines for the Identification and Management of Potential Organ and Tissue Donors*. DH, London. www.dh.gov.uk/en/Publicationsandstatistics/Publications/PublicationsPolicyAndGuidance/DH_4009696 (accessed June 2009).

Department of Health (DH) (2000) *The NHS Cancer Plan*. DH, London. www.dh.gov.uk/en/Publicationsandstatistics/Publications/PublicationsPolicyAndGuidance/DH_4009609 (accessed June 2009).

Department of Health (DH) (2004) *Saving Lives, Valuing Donors: A Transplant Framework for England – One Year on*. DH, London. www.

dh.gov.uk/en/Publicationsandstatistics/Publications/Publications PolicyAndGuidance/DH_4090217 (accessed June 2009).

Department of Health (DH) (2006) *Improving Patients' Access to Medicines: A Guide to Implementing Nurse and Pharmacist Independent Prescribing within the NHS in England*. DH, London. www.dh.gov.uk/en/ Publicationsandstatistics/Publications/PublicationsPolicyAnd Guidance/DH_4133743 (accessed June 2009).

Department of Health (DH) (2008) *End of Life Care Strategy – Promoting High Quality Care for Adults at the End of Life*. Department of Health, London.

Dickman A (2003) Symptom control in care of the dying. In: *Care of the Dying: A Pathway To Excellence* (eds J Ellershaw & S Wilkinson), Oxford University Press, Oxford.

Eliott JA, Olver IA (2007) Do-not-resuscitate orders The implications of dying cancer patients talk on cardiopulmonary resuscitation and do not resuscitate orders. *Qual* Ellershaw J, Ward C (2003) Care of the dying patient: The last hours or days of life. *BMJ* **326**.

Ellershaw J, Wilkinson S (2003) *Care of the Dying: A Pathway to Excellence*. Oxford University Press, Oxford.

Encyclopaedia Britannica (1973) Vol. 5. 15th edn. Encyclopædia Britannica, Inc., Chicago.

Eschun GM, Jacobsohn E, Roberts D, Sniederman B (1999) Ethical and practical considerations of withdrawal of treatment in the intensive care unit. *Can J Anaesthesia* **46**(5): 497–504.

Germain CP (1980) Nursing the dying: Implications of Kübler-Ross staging theory. *Ann Am Acad Political Soc Sci* **447**: 46.

Glare P (2003) Symptom control in care of the dying. In: Ellershaw J & Wilkinson S. *Care of the Dying: A pathway to Excellence*. Oxford University Press, Oxford.

Green J (1993) *Death with Dignity – Meeting the Needs of Patients in a Multi-Cultural Society*. Nursing Times, London.

Higginson I, Sen-Gupta G (2000) Place of care in advanced cancer: a qualitative systematic review of patient preferences. *J Palliat Med* **3**: 287–300.

Howe J (2006) The persistent vegetative state, treatment withdrawal, and the Hillsborough disaster: Airedale NHS Trust v Bland. *Practic Neurol* **6**: 14–27.

Hugel H, Ellershaw J, Gambles M (2006) Respiratory tract secretions in the dying patient: a comparison between glycopyrronium and hyoscine hydrobromide. *J Pall Med* **9**(2): 279–284.

Human Tissue Act (2004) The Stationery Office, London.

Kehl KA (2006) Moving toward peace: An analysis of the concept of a good death. *Am J Hospice Pall Care* **23**: 277.

Kinoshita S (2007) Respecting the wishes of patients in intensive care units. *Nurs Ethics* **14**: 5.

Kübler-Ross E (1969) *On Death and Dying*. Macmillan, New York.

Main J, Whittle C, Treml J, Wolley J, Main A (2006) The development of an Integrated Care Pathway for all patients with advanced life-limiting illness – the supportive care pathway, *J Nurs Man* **14**: 521–528.

Maleck WH, Piper SN, Triem J, Boldt J, Zittel FU (1998) Unexpected return of circulation after cessation of resuscitation (Lazarus phenomenon). *Resuscitation* **39**: 125–128.

Murray S, Kendall M, Boyd K, Tilley S, Ryan D (2004) Spiritual issues and needs: Perspectives from patients with advanced cancer and nonmalignant disease. A qualitative study. *Pall Support Care* **2**: 371–378.

National Council for Palliative Care (2006) *National Survey of Patient Activity Data for Specialist Palliative Care Services Minimum Data Set, Report for the year 2005–2006*. www.ncpc.org.uk/download/mds/MDS_Full_Report_2006.pdf.

National Health Service – End of Life Care Programme (2006) *The Gold Standard Framework: Full Guidance on Using QOF to Improve Palliative/End of Life Care in Primary Care*. www.goldstandardsframework.nhs.uk/content/gp_contract/Full%20Guidance%20on%20Improving%20Palliative%20EOLC%20in%20Primary%20Care%20v25%20July06_1.pdf.

NICE (2004) *Guidance on Cancer Services: Improving Supportive and Palliative Care for Adults with Cancer: The Manual*. NICE, London. www.nice.org.uk/nicemedia/pdf/csgspmanual.pdf.

Office of National Statistics (1999) *1997 Mortality Statistics: General: England and Wales*. The Stationery Office, London.

Office of National Statistics (2004) *Mortality Statistics: Review of the Registrar General on Deaths in England and Wales*. Office for National Statistics, London.

Olsen DP (2007) Arranging live organ donation over the Internet: Is it ethical? Each nurse must decide. *Am J Nurs* **107**: 3.

Price A, Hotopf M, Higginson IJ, Monroe B, Henderson M (2006) Psychological services in hospices in the UK and Republic of Ireland. *J Roy Soc Med* **99**(12): 637–639.

Proulx K, Jacelon C (2004) Dying with dignity: The good patient versus the good death. *Am J Hospice Pall Care* **21**: 116.

Rosseau P (2002) Clinical review article: Non-pain symptom management in the dying patient. *Hosp Physician* 51–56.

Speck P, Higginson I, Addington-Hall J (2004) Spiritual needs in health care may be distinct from religious ones and are integral to palliative care. *BMJ* **329**: 123–124.

Steinhauser KE, Clipp EC, McNeilly M, Christakis MD, McIntyre LM, Tulsky J (2000) In search of a good death: observations of patients, families, and providers. *Ann Intern Med* **132**: 10.

Storey L, Pemberton C, Howard A, O'Donnell LA (2003) Place of death: Hobson's choice or patient choice. *Cancer Nursing Practice* **2**: 33–38.

Thomas K (2003) Community palliative care. In: *The ABC of Palliative Care*, (eds M Fallon & G Hanks), pp. 69–73. Blackwell Publishing, Oxford.

Trovo de Araujo MM, da Silva MJ (2004) Communication with dying patients – perception of intensive care unit nurses in Brazil. *J Clin Nurs* **13**: 143–149.

Turner K, Chye R, Aggarwal G, Philip J, Skeels A, Lickiss JN (1996) Dignity in dying: A preliminary study of patients in the last three days of life. *J Pall Care* **12**(2): 7–13.

Veerbeek L, Zuylen LV, Gambles M, Swart SJ (2006) Audit of the Liverpool Care Pathway for the dying patient in a Dutch cancer hospital. *J Pall Care* **22**(4): 305.

Walton M (2005) It takes a team to choose the most dignified death. *Aust Nurs J* **13**: 2.

Whetstine LM (2007) Bench-to-bedside review: When is dead really dead – on the legitimacy of using neurologic criteria to determine death. *Critl Care* **11**: 208.

Wildiers H, Menten J (2002) Death rattle: prevalence, prevention and treatment. *J Pain Symptom Man* **23**(4): 310–317.

Winter B, Cohen S (1999) ABC of intensive care: Withdrawal of treatment. *BMJ* **319**: 306–308.

Symptom Control at the End of Life

2

Louisa Hunwick, Shareen Juwle and Glen Mitchell

INTRODUCTION

Symptom control is a key component in providing palliative care to patients and their families, but despite the emphasis on the importance of effective management of distressing symptoms, there is considerable evidence that this does not always happen.

Symptoms usually indicate that something is wrong and medical help should be sought. In palliative care, symptoms move beyond being useful indicators of illness to become distressing reminders of advanced disease, which impact in a negative way on quality of life and the ability to function normally in daily activities.

Symptoms are often interlinked and, in palliative care, occur in conjunction with other experiences such as adjusting to changes and losses in role, relationships, independence as well as the concept of facing dying and death (Aranda, 2003).

The aim of this chapter is to provide an overview to symptom control at the end of life.

LEARNING OUTCOMES

At the end of this chapter, the reader will be able to:

❏ Discuss the management of pain.
❏ Describe the management of nausea and vomiting.
❏ Outline the management of bowel obstruction.
❏ Discuss the management of constipation.
❏ Discuss the management of anorexia.
❏ Describe the management of anxiety and depression.
❏ Outline the management of fatigue.

MANAGEMENT OF PAIN

Definition of pain

Approximately 30% patients with a diagnosis of cancer complain of some form of pain, but once the condition becomes terminal, this increases to between 70 and 90% (Schofield *et al.*, 2007).

An expression used widely in the palliative setting is 'pain is what the patient says it is'. Broadly speaking this means that the degree of pain is not assessed by tests using clinical measurements but by the patients' own reports and ability to verbalise their distress.

According to Watson *et al.* (2006), pain has more than one element to its interpretation, involving social, physical, psychological and spiritual aspects of the patient experience. Paz & Seymour (2004) concur that pain is not solely a physical experience but affects every aspect of the patient's life (Figure 2.1).

Consequently, in treating the pain, more than one strategy should be used, including pharmacological intervention and non-

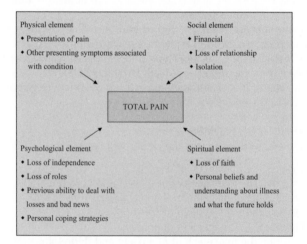

Fig 2.1 Effects of pain on the patient (Adapted from Paz & Seymour 2004)

pharmacological therapies, for example relaxation classes, complementary therapies and anxiety management (Schofield *et al.*, 2007).

Kaye (1994) suggested that pain is the second most common symptom experienced by cancer sufferers. Watson *et al.* (2006) suggested that over 75% of cancer patients identified one or more pain. Twycross concurs by suggesting that over 70% of patients with advanced disease complain of pain; of those patients, 30% complain of a single pain whilst a further 30% experience two types of pain and the remainder experience three or more pains (Twycross, 1997).

Assessment of pain

In order to manage pain successfully a diagnosis and assessment as to the cause of the pain is essential.

Consider:

- Site(s).
- Frequency of pain.
- Duration of pain.
- Loss of power.
- Description of the nature of pain.
- Factors which precipitate pain (e.g. eating, moving).
- Factors which relieve pain.
- Effect of medication on the degree of pain.
- Impact of pain on daily life.
- Whether the pain is continuous.

There are a number of pain assessment questionnaires available that give structure and consistency to history taking. Visual analogue pain charts are of use, enabling patients to score the severity of their pain.

Five key principles have been identified when assessing a patient's pain. It is important to:

- Develop an open relationship with patient and family.
- Allow the patient to talk freely.
- Start with general overall pain questions before homing in on each specific pain.
- Observe for non-verbal indicators of pain.

- Use patient's own words and avoid making assumptions as to how pain presents.

(Watson *et al.*, 2006)

Treatment of pain

In 1986, the World Health Organisation (WHO) published a three-step approach for the relief of cancer-related pain; this later became known worldwide as the 'WHO analgesic ladder' (Figure 2.2).

The WHO analgesic ladder is still considered to be the gold standard for the provision of symptom relief, although it is important to identify that often it is used in a combined approach

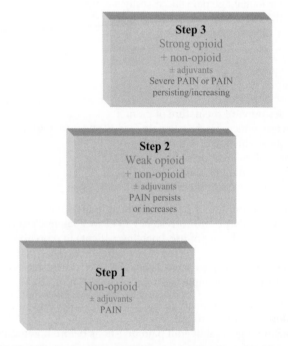

Fig 2.2 World Health Organisation (WHO) analgesic ladder. Reproduced from WHO (1986) *Cancer Pain Relief*, 208, with kind permission of the WHO

with both non-pharmacological therapies and adjuvant analgesics to establish an asymptomatic status. Adjuvant analgesics will be discussed later. Whilst the tool was mainly developed for cancer pain, Stannard & Booth (2004) suggest that it can be applied to chronic pain.

The ladder begins with Step 1 – pain, and suggests 'a non-opioid be given on a regular basis', e.g. paracetamol. If there is no relief or the pain escalates then Step 2 medication is used, i.e. weak opioids should be used either instead of or in conjunction with non-opioids, e.g. codeine, dihydrocodeine. If symptom relief is still not obtained then Step 3 analgesia is required and strong opioids should be administered, e.g. morphine, oxycodone, fentanyl, hydromorphone.

Twycross (1997) recognised that analgesics or co-analgesics from each level of the ladder can be used individually or combined to ensure symptom relief. It is important to stress that the analgesia and level of the patient's pain needs to be reviewed to ensure that the dose is titrated against symptoms to ensure maximum relief (Stannard & Booth, 2004).

The WHO analgesic ladder recommends that medication be administered:

- By the mouth: the oral route is the standard way of administering analgesia, unless the patient's condition dictates otherwise.
- By the clock: pain relief should be administered as a preventative measure on a regular basis.
- By the ladder: the medication should meet the patient's needs. Breakthrough analgesia needs to be in the same potency group as regular analgesia, e.g. a patient on morphine sulphate (slow release) BD should be prescribed Oramorph on an 'as required basis'.

When assessing and addressing pain, it is important to take a multifaceted approach. This incorporates the use of co-analgesics to provide symptom relief. It has long been recognised that there is a place for polypharmacy in pain management (Napp Pharmaceuticals Ltd, 2006). Co-analgesic medication is used when the pain does not completely respond to opioids and is used in conjunction with opioids to augment the symptom relief

(Watson *et al.*, 2006). These co-analgesic medications include corticosteroids and glucocorticoids.

The actions of corticosteroids on the body as a whole are both diverse and complicated. One of the pharmacological responses of glucocorticoids is to reduce inflammation and swelling; pain relief is often achieved by reducing swelling, which provides relief from discomfort and pressure. Whilst the long-term use of steroids is ill advised because of adverse effects, they are commonly used (particularly dexamethasone) to provide symptom relief from pain in palliative care patients (Stannard & Booth, 2004).

Other co-analgesics frequently administered to palliative patients are:

- Non-steroidal anti-inflammatory drugs: useful for bone pain.
- Antispasmodics: for colic.
- Antidepressants: for depression/nerve pain.
- Anticonvulsants: for neuropathic pain.
- Anxiolytics: for anxiety and fear.
- Sedation: for insomnia.

It is essential to address any psychosocial and spiritual aspects of the patient's pain. Worries regarding family, pets, finances and existential factors (e.g. 'why is this happening to me?') may add to the overall painful experience. Basic psychological support may relieve these fears, but patients may need more expert support from a psychologist or chaplain.

Treatment of pain in the dying phase

As the patient's condition deteriorates, the patient may no longer be able to take oral medication. The preferred route for administration of analgesia (usually diamorphine or morphine) is generally subcutaneous, either as a bolus dose or via a syringe driver pump. Other routes of administration such as rectal, intravenous or intramuscular may be impracticable, painful or unacceptable to the patient (Dickman *et al.*, 2005). The syringe driver is a portable infusion device that administers medication continuously over 24 h, providing an effective way of giving symptom relief.

To calculate the dose of analgesia required for the syringe driver, total up the amount of oral morphine sulphate required

Table 2.1 Calculating the correct doses of diamorphine and morphine for use in the syringe driver

Oral morphine sulphate dose (e.g. Zomorph) 15 mg BD = 30 mg 24 h
Subcutaneous dose diamorphine for syringe driver
30 ÷ 3 (24 h total amount of oral morphine) = 10 mg diamorphine in syringe driver
Subcutaneous dose morphine for syringe driver
30 ÷ 2 (total 24 h amount of oral morphine) = 15 mg morphine sulphate in syringe driver

over the previous 24 h, including rescue doses, and divide this by three for the approximate equivalent dose of subcutaneous diamorphine or by two for the approximate equivalent dose of subcutaneous morphine sulphate (Table 2.1) (West Midlands Palliative Care Physicians, 2007). Diamorphine is usually preferable to morphine for subcutaneous opioid administration because it is more soluble (West Midlands Palliative Care Physicians, 2007).

Recognition needs to be given to the importance of providing the correct end-of-life management in order to address the needs of patients and their families. The NHS end-of-life care initiative formulated three programmes/pathways to ensure best practice and improve care received by the terminally ill and their families (National Council for Palliative Care, 2006).

The Liverpool Care Pathway was developed to apply hospice standards in other settings, i.e. hospitals. It promotes consistency in the care of the dying, multidisciplinary care, planning and decision-making, and good communication between the patient, family and staff. It is designed to be used in the last few of days of life and incorporates anticipatory planning for symptom management (including pain, nausea and vomiting, agitation and excess respiratory tract secretions).

Pain in patients with advanced disease can be complex and patients may experience both acute and chronic syndromes associated with the disease. Whilst pharmacological intervention is the first choice for symptom management, it should be used in conjunction with non-drug therapies in order to enhance the pharmacological inputs and gain maximum symptom relief to the patient.

MANAGEMENT OF NAUSEA AND VOMITING

Nausea and vomiting are symptoms that can cause patients and their families and carers deep distress. It is estimated that 50–60% of patients with advanced cancer will suffer from it (Baines, 1997). Many patients can often tolerate one or two episodes of vomiting a day but prolonged nausea is very debilitating (Watson *et al.*, 2006).

Linking nausea and vomiting together is in some ways unfortunate, as many people regard nausea as synonymous with vomiting. This is not always the case, although there is an obvious connection between the two. Nausea does not always result in vomiting and vomiting can be sudden and not preceded by feelings of nausea, therefore they should be regarded as two separate phenomena.

Nausea is an unpleasant sensation that may precede vomiting and is associated with signs of increased activity of the sympathetic nervous system, i.e. tachycardia, increased salvation and sweating. It is very subjective and can be more prolonged and less easily controlled than vomiting. Nausea disturbs the normal pattern of the motility of the gut (a regular rhythm of contraction and relaxation) by causing a slowing and sometimes complete cessation of gastric motility (gastric stasis). This prevents further digestion of food; toxins are absorbed and retroperistalsis occurs (moving contents from the duodenum into the stomach ready for expulsion by vomiting) (Hawthorn, 1995).

Vomiting is described as the forceful expulsion of gastric contents through the mouth and is thought to be a primitive protective mechanism against ingesting toxic or harmful substances (Kaye, 1994). Vomiting is a complex process, which is controlled by the vomiting centre in the brain. This is stimulated by a variety of pathways that originate from the chemoreceptor trigger zone (CTZ), the vestibular apparatus, the cerebral cortex and the abdominal viscera (Figure 2.3) (Millership, 2003).

Causes of nausea and vomiting

It is important to understand the cause(s) of nausea and vomiting (Tables 2.2a–c) in order to offer the most appropriate treatment to the patient.

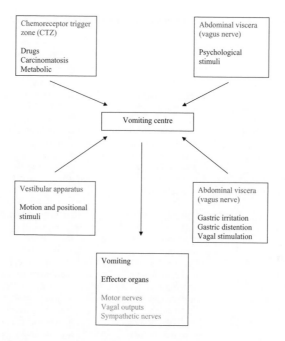

Fig 2.3 Detectors and effectors of the need to vomit (Adapted from Millership, 2003 and Twycross, 1997)

Assessment of the patient

Assessment is vital to identify and treat the cause as quickly as possible in order to gain the confidence of the patient. Twycross (1999) suggests that it is usually possible to determine the cause from the patient's history and a clinical examination. Aranda (2003) defines assessment of symptoms as systematic attention to the physical, emotional, social and spiritual impact of advanced disease. It is important to assess:

- The nature of the symptom, i.e. timing, duration and severity.
- The level of discomfort it causes, i.e. what effect it has on daily life, how distressing it is.
- The patient's understanding, i.e. concerns, fears, expectations of what it means in terms of their illness.

Table 2.2a Causes of nausea and vomiting: gastrointestinal tract (Adapted from Kaye, 1994)

Cause	Features	Treatment
Oral thrush	White plaques	Ketoconazole,
Gastric irritation	Indigestion, reflux, drugs,	fluconazole, nystatin
Squashed stomach	e.g. NSAIDs, steroids	H_2 inhibitor, PPI, stop or
syndrome	Hiccoughs, heartburn,	change NSAID
Gastric outflow	early satiety, epigastric	Small meals antacids,
obstruction	fullness, heartburn,	H_2 inhibitor, pro-kinetic
Gastric stasis	nausea on eating,	anti-emetic, e.g.
Ascites	small volume vomiting	metoclopramide
Bowel obstruction	Large volume vomits,	Steroids, octreotide (if
Constipation	every 1–2 days, little	persistent)
	nausea	Pro-kinetic anti-emetic,
	Large volume vomit –	e.g. metoclopramide
	reflux. Relieves nausea	Paracentesis (if
	Abdominal distension and	appropriate)
	discomfort	Spironolactone
	Large volume, projectile	Surgery (if appropriate)
	vomiting may be	Medical management:
	faeculent	stop laxatives and
	Abdominal pain – may be	pro-kinetic anti-emetics
	distension	Syringe driver with
	Constipation/diarrhoea	diamorphine/morphine
	Abdominal discomfort,	sulphate and
	bowels not opened for	Buscopan cyclizine or
	several days	octreotide
	Sometimes nausea	Laxatives, enema PR if
		appropriate

NSAID, non-steroidal anti-inflammatory drug; PPI, protein pump inhibitor; PR, per rectum

Table 2.2b Causes of nausea and vomiting: cerebral (Adapted from Kaye, 1994)

Cause	Features	Treatment
Anxiety/fear	Nausea ('sick with fear')	Anxiolytics, counselling
Brain metastases	Patient may not	explanation
	recognise anxiety	High-dose steroids, e.g.
	Anti-emetics are not	dexamethasone 12–16 mg
	effective	daily. Refer to oncologist
	Headaches, projectile	re radiotherapy
	vomiting, neurological	
	signs, little nausea	

Table 2.2c Causes of nausea and vomiting: metabolic (Adapted from Kaye, 1994)

Cause	Features	Treatment
Hypercalcaemia	Drowsiness, confusion	Hydration (intravenous)
Uraemia	Hiccoughs, twitching confusion, drowsiness	Bisphosphonates, e.g. disodium pamidronate IV
		Explanation, sedation, e.g. midazolam (sub-cutaneously)
Cough	Retching/vomiting after coughing, little nausea	Tissues, nebuliser (saline) antibiotics
UTI	Offensive urine, frequency incontinence	MSU/CSU for culture and sensitivity
Drugs, e.g. opiates, antibiotics, digoxin, iron	Nausea; question if symptom is linked to when drug started	Antibiotics Stop or reduce drug Add anti-emetic to opiate

IV, intravenous; UTI, urinary tract infection; MSU, midstream specimen of urine; CSU, catheter specimen of urine

- Previous experiences or fears of possible outcomes of reporting symptoms, e.g. disease progression, hospitalisation (Hill, 2006).

Assessment of nausea and vomiting involves taking a detailed history of the pattern, speed of onset and precipitating factors (Kaye, 1994). Ask about:

- Timing and frequency of vomits.
- Relationship to food, drugs, other experiences.
- Amounts, projectile, reflux, faeculent.
- Is nausea present?
- Does vomiting relieve nausea?
- Any other symptoms, e.g. pain, vertigo?
- How does it interfere with daily life?
- Ability to eat and drink.
- Effect of previously tried anti-emetics – doses, route.

  Physical examination should include:

- Abdominal examination for masses, ascites, epigastric tenderness/rebound, hepatomegaly, constipation, abnormal/absent bowel sounds.

- Close patient observation for signs of dehydration, jaundice, papilloedema, thrush, neurological signs (Hill, 2006).

Decisions on the relevance of continuing invasive investigations are based on the history, clinical examination, illness trajectory and intention to intervene. At the end stage of illness when death is close, investigations are unlikely to add value to the management and can be counterproductive in the provision of good palliative care (Millership, 2003).

Treatment of nausea and vomiting

Treatment of nausea and vomiting is based on blocking the effects of specific neurotransmitters in the brain and the gut by using drugs that act as antagonists on receptors (Table 2.3).

Before choosing an anti-emetic:

- Determine the possible cause(s) of nausea and vomiting.
- Treat any reversible causes.
- Review current medication.
- Ensure the patient understands and agrees with the treatment plan.

(Thompson, 2004)

Table 2.3 Receptor blockade by anti-emetics (adapted from Kaye, 2003)

	Chemoreceptor trigger zone	Vomiting centre	Gut wall
Receptors	D2 5HT2	H1 Cholin	5HT3 5HT4
Metoclopramide	++		+ ++
Haloperidol	+++		
Cyclizine		++ ++	
Levomepromazine	++ +++	+++ ++	
Granisetron			+++
Hyoscine hydrobromide			

To use an anti-emetic effectively:

- Choose an anti-emetic based on its specific mode of action; first- and second-line anti-emetics are listed in Tables 2.4 and 2.5.
- Choose the most appropriate route of administration; oral anti-emetics are only effective in preventing nausea or treating mild nausea. For the control of nausea or vomiting, anti-emetics need to be administered via an injection (intramuscular or subcutaneous) or a suppository. This is because nausea causes gastric stasis and prevents absorption of oral drugs. See Table 2.6 for routes of administration.

Table 2.4 First-line anti-emetics (Adapted from Kaye, 2003; West Midlands Palliative Care Physicians, 2007)

Cause	Drug
Gastric stasis	Metoclopramide
Gastric irritation	10–20 mg TDS PO
Partial/pseudo bowel obstruction	30–100 mg/24 h CSCI
Drug induced	Haloperidol
Biochemical	1.5–3 mg OD PO
Metabolic	1.5–10 mg/24 h CSCI
Bowel obstruction (complete)	Cyclizine (can be 50 mg TDS PO
Raised intracranial pressure	combined with 150 mg/24 h CSCI
Motion related	haloperidol)

OD, once daily; PO, orally; CSCI, continuous subcutaneous infusion; TDS, three times daily

Table 2.5 Second-line anti-emetics (Adapted from Kaye, 2003; West Midlands Palliative Care Physicians, 2007)

Cause	Drug
Broad spectrum anti-emetic which acts on several receptors; therefore can cover many causes of nausea and vomiting	Levomepromazine 6.25 mg OD PO (¼ of 25 mg tablet) 6.25–25 mgs/24 h CSCI
Chemically induced bowel obstruction	Dexamethasone 4–16 mg OD PO
Raised intracranial pressure	4–16 mg/24 h CSCI (adjuvant – increases the effect of other drugs)

OD, once daily; PO, orally; CSCI, continuous subcutaneous infusion

Table 2.6 Routes for administration of anti-emetics

Continuous sub-cutaneous infusion (CSCI)	Via a syringe driver is the most effective route to use for nausea and vomiting; particularly suited to palliative care as it is simple, safe and minimally intrusive to the patient
Intramuscular	Should be avoided unless absolutely necessary as it is likely to be painful, particularly for the cachexic patient
Intravenous infusion	Not always appropriate (or possible) as venous access can be difficult to obtain
Rectal administration	Invasive and sometimes painful or distressing for the terminally ill patient

- Ensure regular and maximum dose of anti-emetic is tried before changing to another.
- Avoid using drugs with anticholinergic effects, e.g. hyoscine, cyclizine in patients with gastric stasis.
- Do not administer an anticholinergic drug, e.g. cyclizine, concurrently with a pro-kinetic drug, e.g. metoclopramide, because it could antagonise the effects of the latter.
- Try an alternative drug if the first anti-emetic prescribed is ineffective (if only partially effective, add another anti-emetic, e.g. haloperidol, added to cyclizine).
- Review the patient on a regular basis to monitor the effectiveness of the treatment.

(West Midlands Palliative Care Physicians, 2007).

Non-drug measures include:

- Calm, reassuring environment away from the sight and smell of food or unpleasant odours.
- Avoid exposure to foods that precipitate nausea.
- Give small amounts of food more often.
- Complementary therapies.
- Regular mouth care.

MANAGEMENT OF BOWEL OBSTRUCTION

Bowel obstruction at the end stage of the disease process can be caused by several factors. It most commonly occurs with cancer of the ovary or bowel and can be caused by intrinsic or extrinsic pressure by either a primary tumour or metastatic abdominal and/or pelvic disease. Other causes are from previous treatments such as post-radiation therapy, adhesions from previous surgery, unrelated conditions such as a strangulated hernia, severe constipation or a combination of factors.

Obstruction can be mechanical, functional or both, affecting single or multiple sites, partial or complete, high, low or both, and transient or persistent (Twycross, 1997; Watson *et al.*, 2006). Surgical intervention should only be considered in advanced disease if an easily reversible cause seems likely, e.g. local, single obstruction or adhesions and the patient's general condition is good, e.g. independent and active, and is willing to undergo surgery.

It is contra-indicated if intra-abdominal carcinomatosis is evident, recurrent ascites despite paracentesis, or evidence from previous laparotomy that successful intervention will not be likely. The potential mortality and morbidity associated with surgery must be weighed against quality of life for a patient with a prognosis of weeks (Watson *et al.*, 2006).

If surgical intervention is inappropriate, management of symptoms using medication can generally be very effective and the use of a nasogastric tube and intravenous fluids (drip and suck) need rarely be used.

Symptoms of bowel obstruction often arise gradually over a period of time rather than with a sudden onset. There may be a history of constipation with colic, followed by poor appetite, fatigue, increased nausea with eventual vomiting. Following on from these symptoms there may be intermittent abdominal pain, abdominal distension and a reduction or complete absence of bowel sounds (Thompson, 2004).

However, there can be variations from the classic symptoms, with little abdominal distension if widespread tumour infiltration has occurred. It may be episodic, with symptoms occurring for a few days then settling, and there may be intermittent diarrhoea with constipation (Kaye, 1994). Radiological investigations are helpful to distinguish the cause and help to identify whether surgical intervention is a suitable option.

Medical treatment of bowel obstruction

The aim of medical treatment is to control symptoms so that quality of life can be maximised by enabling patients to eat and drink to their own limits.

It is unlikely that medications will be absorbed in the gut, therefore they should be administered by continuous subcutaneous infusion using a syringe driver. If the obstruction is incomplete (passing flatus and no colic), a prokinetic drug, e.g. metoclopramide, which increases gastric emptying and reduces gastric volume, should be used in combination with dexamethasone. This may help to reduce oedema around the obstruction site, potentially increasing the patency of the lumen of the bowel as well as having an anti-emetic effect. However, when complete bowel obstruction is present, a prokinetic anti-emetic increases colic and dexamethasone increases gastric acid production, causing the patient further discomfort and this is therefore not indicated for use (Baines, 1998).

If colic is present, discontinue bulk-forming, osmotic and stimulating laxatives. Vomiting is often the most difficult symptom to control and in some patients it has to be acknowledged that they may continue to vomit once or twice a day despite best efforts to control with drugs. Drugs used to control vomiting include:

- Cyclizine 150 mg/24 h via continuous subcutaneous infusion (syringe driver). Haloperidol can be added if nausea persists, 1.5–5 mg/24 h.
- Levomepromazine 6.25–25 mg/24 h is a broad-spectrum anti-emetic, which is very useful as second-line anti-emetic. It also has sedative effects, which may be welcomed by the patient during the last few days of life.
- Hyoscine butylbromide 60–120 mg/24 h. Reduces or encourages reabsorption of intestinal secretions and reduces gut motility.
- Octreotide 250–1000 mcg/24 h is a somatostatin analogue and has similar antisecretory properties as hyoscine butylbromide with no anticholinergic effects. However, it is very expensive but has a fast action and high efficacy (Watson *et al.*, 2006).

If the patient is experiencing constant background pain diamorphine/morphine sulphate should be administered appropriately via a syringe driver over 24 h.

A nasogastric tube and intravenous fluids can be very invasive and distressing for the patient and are rarely necessary to control symptoms in bowel obstruction. However, some patients, for whom vomiting is considered wholly unacceptable, might prefer the option of a nasogastric tube and intravenous fluids; it is therefore important to consider patient choice and discuss the options with them.

If possible, patients should be encouraged to eat and drink to their own limits. The use of anticholinergic drugs and diminished fluids can often cause dry mouth; this can be managed successfully by attention to good regular mouth care (Twycross, 1997).

MANAGEMENT OF CONSTIPATION

Constipation is defined as the difficult or incomplete defecation of hard stools less frequently than the individual's normal bowel action (Anderson *et al.*, 1994). Faecal impaction can occur if constipation continues without treatment, extending as far back as the caecum. This can lead to faecal overflow, diarrhoea and leakage. This is often mistaken for diarrhoea and may be treated with anti-diarrhoeal drugs such as loperamide, which will then compound the problem.

Causes of constipation

Causes of constipation in patients with advanced disease include:

- Poor fluid intake: lack of thirst can lead to dehydration; this leads to more fluid being absorbed from the colon, which is the body's mechanism to balance hydration.
- Poor nutrition: reduced dietary fibre reduces the ability of the stool to retain fluid.
- Reduced mobility: lack of exercise decreases bowel motility.
- Painful bowel action: due to prolapsed haemorrhoids, anal fissure or rectal tumour.
- Drugs, e.g. opioids, anticholinergics, diuretics; opioids are the most commont cause of severe constipation.

- Inability to access toilet facilities unaided.
- Difficult toileting, e.g. using bedpan rather than toilet/commode (Kaye, 1994; Regnard *et al.*, 2004; Watson *et al.*, 2006)).
- Hypercalcaemia.

Treatment of constipation

Ideally, constipation should be prevented but in reality that is extremely difficult to achieve because of the nature of the causes. Patients who are terminally ill are generally not able to follow the advice or treatment offered to other patients suffering from constipation, i.e. increase fluid intake and fibre in diet and encourage exercise/mobility. Dying patients rarely experience thirst or hunger, therefore eating and drinking are no longer priorities and may even become a burden. Intravenous fluids are rarely necessary unless the patient complains of thirst and often this can be resolved by offering regular mouth care and sips of fluid (Kaye, 1994).

Measures that can be taken to reduce the incidence of constipation for these patients include:

- Stopping or reducing any medication that is not essential for symptom control.
- Responding to requests for toileting in a timely manner with the appropriate facility, e.g. take the patient into the toilet if possible to allow privacy, dignity and correct positioning to open bowels more easily.
- Always prescribing an appropriate laxative with analgesics that are known to cause constipation, i.e. opioids, codeine, hyoscine.
- Administering laxatives (see below) on a regular basis, using an effective dose and monitor the result daily by using a stool chart, e.g. Bristol stool form scale (Lewis & Heaton, 1997).
- Performing *per rectum* examination (if appropriate) to assess the need for suppository/enema, i.e. is the rectum full of faeces? What is the consistency?
- Offering a suppository or enema as appropriate.

Laxatives are divided into four categories:

- Stimulants, e.g. senna, dantron, bisacodyl.
- Osmotic agents, e.g. lactulose, macrogol preparations, e.g. Movicol. Macrogols are inert polymers of ethylene glycol, which retain fluid in the bowel; taking fluid with macrogols may reduce the dehydrating effect sometimes seen with osmotic laxatives (Martin & Mehta, 2007).
- Bulk-forming agents, e.g. fibrogel, normacol and methylcellulose, are not recommended for use in palliative/terminal care as they are likely to worsen constipation when fluid intake is poor; they need to be consumed very quickly because the preparation sets within minutes of being mixed, and this is likely to be beyond capabilities of the terminally ill patient.
- Faecal softeners, e.g. docusate, are useful when combined with a stimulant (docusate and dantron = co-danthrusate, docusate and poloxamer = co-danthramer); combination preparations help to keep medications to a minimum.

When choosing a laxative, the following needs to be considered:

- Patient choice and/or ability to take may dictate/limit choice.
- Osmotic agents may not be suitable to use in the terminally ill patient as it is recommended to drink 2–3l of water to maximise their effect; in addition it can cause flatulence and abdominal cramps.
- Stimulant drugs should be avoided if there is a possibility of intestinal obstruction.
- Senna has a greater tendency to cause colic than dantron/combination laxative.

MANAGEMENT OF ANOREXIA

Anorexia (and the associated malnutrition) is a common symptom in terminal patients and can be difficult to manage. Bruera & MacDonald (1988) found that malnutrition occurred in 51% of patients with advanced disease and 80% of patients in the terminal stages of their disease. They list three main causes of malnutrition: decreased nutritional intake, increased need for calories and malabsorption.

Meares (2000) describes irreversible malnutrition as 'cancer anorexia – cachexia syndrome'. This is where the patient suffers from anorexia, tissue wasting and poor functional status, eventually leading to death. When a person reaches this stage, it is rarely reversible.

Assessment of the patient

When assessing patients with poor appetite, it is important to find out why they do not wish to eat. There may be treatable causes, which can be addressed so that it improves their appetite (see Box 2.1). There can be multiple causes for anorexia, making this a multifaceted symptom. Therefore, a thorough holistic assessment is required to identify all aspects of the patient's anorexia.

Treatment of anorexia

Some medications that stimulate appetite can be used alongside non-pharmacological methods (see Box 2.2). For example, a low-dose steroid such as dexamethasone can be effective, although it is important to note that long-term use of steroids can diminish their effect of stimulating appetite.

Less commonly, megesterol acetate can be used to temporarily stimulate the appetite; the advantage of this drug is that it can be used for a few months. It can cause bloating and masculinisation and may not be acceptable for some patients.

Box 2.1 Treatable causes of anorexia

- Pain.
- Mouth conditions including dryness, gum soreness and infections such as oral candidiasis.
- Constipation.
- Reflux oesophagitis.
- Nausea and vomiting.
- Ascites.
- Difficulty swallowing.
- Anxiety.
- Biochemical – hypercalcaemia, hyponatraemia and uraemia.
- Treatments, e.g. drugs, radiotherapy, chemotherapy.

Box 2.2 Non-pharmacological methods of treating anorexia

- Offer small high-calorie meals.
- Offer meals on smaller plates so that patients do not feel they have to eat large meals. Sometimes large meals can induce nausea.
- Having a glass of wine before meals can stimulate the appetite.
- Offer supplementary drinks in between meals to increase calorie intake.
- Seek advice from a dietician for other high-calorie meals/drinks for the patient and to provide advice to patients regarding their appetite.
- If patients require anti-emetics ensure they are given at least half an hour prior to meals.
- Allow patients to eat foods that they desire whenever they wish. In hospitals, the family should be encouraged to bring in foods which the patient wants if it cannot be obtained within the hospital.
- Explore/address emotional and spiritual issues, which may impact on the patient's weight loss.

Sometimes intravenous fluids or parenteral feeding may be required. When considering other forms of feeding, it is important to include the wishes of the patients in the decision-making process. The impact on their quality of life should be considered and issues surrounding altered body image should be explored with them.

Patients who have difficulty swallowing, e.g. due to tumour invasion from an oesophageal cancer, may require another form of feeding in order to maintain or increase their nutritional intake; nasogastric feeding, percutaneous endoscopic gastrostomy feeding or total parenteral nutrition intravenously are three non-oral methods of feeding. However, it is important to acknowledge that if patients are in the dying phase of their illness, these invasive procedures may not be in their best interests because they can prolong life.

Artificial hydration, such as intravenous or subcutaneous fluids, remain an ethical subject. As with parenteral feeding, the continuation or commencement of these interventions may not be in the best interests of the patient. Twycross & Wilcock (2001) state that artificial hydration should not be introduced to satisfy the wishes of relatives. The family members and the patient should be given reasons for this in a sensitive manner.

Nutrition at the end of life

Loss of appetite can often be a sign of advancing disease and an indicator that a person is nearing the end of life, as the desire for food and drink lessens (Thornes & Garrard, 2003). At the end of life, nutritional care should be focused on alleviating symptoms and satisfying the patient's comfort needs.

This can be a distressing time for the patient and more so for the relatives. Relatives often worry that their loved one is not eating and may put pressure on them to eat more (which could increase the patient's distress). Sometimes the patient may seek permission to eat less and it is important for nurses to give this permission to enable the patient to have reassurance and be at ease.

The patient and their relatives should be reassured that anorexia and a reduced appetite is normal at the end of life and that 'force feeding' and artificial hydration is ineffective at this stage and will not prolong life but instead may cause more discomfort with greater risks of 'overloading' the patient with fluids.

It is important to re-iterate that when caring for terminal patients, the focus is put on alleviating any symptoms. Although patients may not wish to eat they may enjoy a refreshing drink to their liking or to keep their mouth and lips moist. It can be helpful to allow relatives to give this care by giving regular sips of fluid or teaching them to use mouth care swabs or sponges, to allow them to be involved in the care and feel they are maintaining their loved one's comfort.

Conversely, patients who are kept nil by mouth who are at the end of life may want to eat/drink and become distressed when not able to do so. As comfort measures are important at this time, it may be necessary to allow the patient to have small amounts of food and drink to chew and expel or swallow to maintain their comfort despite the risk of aspiration. This decision should be made by healthcare professionals agreeing that it is in the patient's best interests and that the patient's comfort needs are being met.

MANAGEMENT OF ANXIETY AND DEPRESSION

Anxiety and depression are unpleasant emotions that are distressing for patients and can be difficult for healthcare professionals to manage. These symptoms remain under-diagnosed and under-treated in palliative care patients since they are often thought of as an understandable or normal reaction to an incurable illness (Barraclough, 1997). They are usually reactions to losses and threats of the illness such as loss of role, uncertainty and fears of death and dying. The risk factors for these symptoms are similar and can impact on each other.

Risk factors for anxiety and depression

Risk factors for anxiety and depression include:

- Poorly controlled physical symptoms such as severe pain.
- Social isolation or lack of social support.
- History of mood disorders/alcohol or substance abuse.
- Difficult relationships and communications between staff and patients.
- Family history or past history of depression.

(Barraclough, 1997)

Anxiety

Kaye (1994) describes anxiety as a state of apprehension or fear. It can be acute or chronic and can vary in intensity. Anxiety can be caused by many factors and impinge upon any symptoms that the patient may already have, such as breathlessness. Therefore, it is important to identify and manage symptoms holistically. Caution should be taken when making too many changes to the management of any symptoms and should be limited to one or two changes at a time, as effects of these changes on the patient's symptoms will be more difficult to identify. Signs and symptoms of anxiety are listed in Table 2.7.

Table 2.7 Signs and symptoms of anxiety (Adapted from Barraclough 1997 and Mitten, 2006)

• Agitation	• Nausea
• Panic	• Urinary frequency/diarrhoea
• Restlessness	• Headaches
• Shortness of breath	• Worry
• Dizziness	• Inability to relax
• Sweating	• Difficulty concentrating
• Nightmares	• Difficulty sleeping
• Apprehension	• Irritability
• Muscular aches	• Palpitations
• Dry mouth	

Table 2.8 Signs and symptoms of depression (Adapted from Barraclough, 1997)

• Withdrawn	• Delusions
• Tearful	• Expressionless face
• Quiet	• Reduced energy, fatigue
• Disturbed sleep, early wakening	• Reduced concentration
• Anorexia, diminished appetite	• Low mood
• Feeling as if life is worthless	• Indecisiveness
• Low self esteem	• Pessimistic ideas about the future
• Lack of interest	• Suicidal thoughts or acts

Depression

Mitten (2006) describes depression as low mood or low self-esteem for at least two weeks. Throughout the patients' illness, such as at the time of diagnosis or relapses, they may present with psychological distress such as low mood, fear, sadness or anger. These are recognised as adjustment reactions, which can cause distressing emotions and present as depression for a short period of time. Usually they resolve within a few weeks with support from the patient's family, friends and professionals involved in their care. It is therefore important to reassess the patient in order to differentiate between an adjustment reaction and a depressive state. Signs and symptoms of depression are listed in Table 2.8.

Non-pharmacological treatment for anxiety and depression

The non-pharmacological management for anxiety and depression is similar. It is important to note that, as with all symptoms discussed in this chapter, a holistic assessment of the patient should be undertaken. This enables the nurse to develop a therapeutic relationship with patients and identify how their symptoms affect each other.

One of the simplest and most important methods that nurses can provide for the management of anxiety and depression is to listen to the concerns and issues of the patient. This in itself can be reassuring to the patient and may relieve acute symptoms such as panic or restlessness. It is vital to be sensitive and non-judgemental when listening to the patient's concerns. Patients should have the opportunity to express their feelings without fear of being abandoned (Barraclough, 1997), therefore nurses should allow enough time for the patients to discuss their concerns and be allowed to express their emotions openly.

Referrals to other members of the multidisciplinary team can be helpful, such as the palliative care team, to provide extra support to the patient and advice to the nursing and medical team. If patients have spiritual or religious distress that is impacting on their symptoms or if the patient finds relief in religion or prayer, it may be necessary to involve other professionals such as chaplains to help the patient and in turn reduce the severity of the symptoms.

Educating relatives and the patient to help themselves in acute situations can be helpful and instil a sense of control. For example, teaching deep breathing and relaxation methods could help in acute anxiety or panic attacks. With permission from the patient, complementary therapies such as massage, reflexology, aromatherapy and reiki can be offered in order to promote a sense of calm and control. Indications for referral to a psychologist include:

- If the patient is extremely withdrawn.
- If the patient expresses suicidal thoughts or acts.
- Previous psychiatric history.
- Symptoms persist despite attempts to treat them.

Pharmacological treatment for anxiety and depression
Drugs used for anxiety include the following.

Benzodiazepines

Effective for anxiety and are better if limited to short term or intermittent use as prolonged use can reduce the anxiolytic effect. They do not remove the anxiety from a patient but simply suppress it (Twycross & Wilcock, 2001), therefore non-pharmacological methods should be used concurrently (see above). Two commonly use benzodiazepines:

- Lorazepam 0.5–1 mg tds/prn sublingual/oral: a short-acting drug useful for anxiety or panic attacks if given sublingually (faster onset).
- Diazepam 2–5 mg tds/nocte (increase according to response): longer acting than lorazepam and is particularly useful for muscle relaxation.

Antipsychotic drugs

- Haloperidol 1.5–10 mg daily oral/subcutaneously: more effective in patients with an element of confusion or paranoia; caution must be taken in the elderly (lower doses should be prescribed).

Tricyclic antidepressants

- Amitriptyline 10–25 mg oral at night initially (can be increased to 50 mg): effective for panic disorders and when depression is present. It can take up to several weeks to have full effect.

(Back, 2001)

When patients are in the dying phase, the treatment for anxiety or terminal restlessness is different. Terminal restlessness is an overwhelming anxiety, not amenable to reassurance (Barraclough, 1997), and its features are being unable to relax physically, twitching and calling out (Flynn & Quinn, 2003). It can be distressing for the family to witness this, therefore the needs of the family should be acknowledged and reassured. In terminal restlessness, it is effective to use benzodiazepines such as midazolam 2.5–5 mg subcutaneously stat as it has a sedating, anticonvulsant and anxiolytic effect. The dose should then be titrated to what the patient requires over a 24-h period and administered subcutaneously via a continuous syringe driver. The aim is to keep patients rousable.

However, in order to keep patients comfortable at the end of life, sedation is often needed (Flynn & Quinn, 2003).

Drugs used for depression are specific serotonin reuptake inhibitors (SSRI):

- Citalopram 10–20 mg oral tds (maximum 60 mg daily)
- Sertraline 50 mg oral daily
- Paroxetine 20 mg oral daily.

(Kaye, 1992; Back, 2001)

These are non-sedative and are safer in overdose. However, they can cause nausea, diarrhoea, headaches and anxiety:

It is important that pharmacological and non-pharmacological methods are used alongside each other in order to provide effective symptom management for anxiety and depression. If the patient's symptoms persist despite these interventions, it is vital to seek specialist psychiatric support.

MANAGEMENT OF FATIGUE

Fatigue is the most common symptom encountered by patients with advanced disease, with approximately 75–90% of patients experiencing it (Ross & Alexander, 2001). According to Carpentino (1995, in Porock, 2003) fatigue is defined as 'an overwhelming, sustained sense of exhaustion and decreased capacity for physical and mental work that is not relieved by rest'. Common signs and symptoms of fatigue are listed in Box 2.3.

Fatigue can occur at anytime during the dying process and fluctuate throughout. Unfortunately fatigue can be under-diagnosed, although it is a common symptom. Little is known about how it develops and it can sometimes be overlooked (Ahlberg *et al.*, 2003), therefore the treatment for fatigue may be unsuccessful.

The causes of fatigue can be physical, as part of the disease process, psychological, for example from anxiety and depression, and result from treatments such as medications, surgery, chemotherapy and radiotherapy (Porock, 2003). It is important to recognise that fatigue can be multifaceted and have more than one causative factor.

Fatigue can be distressing for patients as it can impair their quality of life and impinge on their sense of well-being, daily

---

Box 2.3 Common signs and symptoms of fatigue

- Tiredness.
- Lack of energy.
- Weakness.
- Boredom.
- Lethargy.
- Exhaustion.
- Lack of motivation.
- Inability to concentrate.
- Depression.
- Loss.
- Psychological stress.

---

performance, activities of daily living, relationships and general mood. It is a total experience affecting the patient physically, mentally, emotionally and socially. It is therefore important for the nurse to identify what factors may be causing the fatigue and how it is affecting the patient in order to help with the symptoms.

Assessment of fatigue

When trying to assess and manage fatigue, the nurse should approach the patient in a sensitive manner. Ross & Alexander (2001) suggest that a thorough nursing assessment of the patient is required and should include identifying factors which exacerbate or help to relieve fatigue, identify how the patient's activities of daily living are affected and establish the potential causes of fatigue.

It is important to address all factors contributing to fatigue. The management of fatigue as a single symptom is not enough to control alone (Porock, 2003). Other symptoms that the patient experiences should also be assessed as these may affect or intensify the fatigue. For example, if a patient has uncontrolled pain or emotional distress they are likely to have an effect on each other and the patient's overall fatigue. It is therefore vital to address and manage these other symptoms in order to also impact on the fatigue.

Patients who experience fatigue may sense a loss of control, which could impinge further on their quality of life. Patients should be empowered to maintain control over any decisions regarding their care and assist them to understand and find meaning in their fatigue (Lane, 2005). This can be achieved by providing the patient and their families with education and information about fatigue and its management. Porock (2003) suggests that if this is done earlier in the patients' journey, it can prevent unnecessary distress as they will know what to expect and it gives control back to the patient.

Treatment of fatigue

The patient needs to be educated on strategies to help manage fatigue. It is essential to note that rest alone cannot relieve fatigue and the nurse needs to aid patients in finding a balance between activity and rest to ensure that their energy is used effectively. Skalla & Lacasse (1992) describe conserving and using energy in this way as an energy bank. Energy is saved by rest and extra nutrition, and is spent on doing tasks that require more energy.

Complementary therapies may help some patients with symptoms of fatigue. According to Fellowes *et al.* (2004, in Lane, 2005) there is evidence to show relaxation, massage and aromatherapy can benefit patients with depression and fatigue. Medications such as corticosteroids and psycho-stimulants can be beneficial in treating fatigue, but the effects of these drugs may decline after a period of time (Ross & Alexander, 2001).

If the patient is feeling more fatigued and sleepy it may be a sign that the end of life is near (Porock, 2003). It is imperative to continue communicating with the patient and their families and to explain that this is a normal process. Some patients may seek to be given 'permission' to rest.

When considering the use of drugs to treat patients at the end of life, their comfort and wishes should take priority. Taking medications that will not prolong their life or benefit their outcome should not be used at this stage as it may be more distressing for them. For example, taking oral steroids may mean taking a lot of tablets; imposing this on patients may increase their distress further.

The comfort and best wishes of the patient should be of importance at the end of life, and strategies of managing fatigue may not be of any benefit, but maintaining communication and supporting the patient and their relatives will make their experience less distressing.

CONCLUSION

There comes a stage when dying patients begin to lose interest in everyday events and activities around them. At this time the nursing staff need to be clear about the goals of care and help families and friends to understand the dying process. Recognition needs to be given to the importance of keeping families informed of any changes and giving them the opportunity to be involved in decisions about the care of their loved one (O'Connor, 2003).

The focus of care for dying patients is to manage their symptoms to a level that is acceptable to them without compromising quality of life. It is also important to enable the patient to deal with any unfinished business should they so wish.

Good control of symptoms is vital in the last days of life to ensure a peaceful death for the patient and positive memories for their families and friends who live on without them (Millership, 2003). The professional's sensitive and compassionate care of the terminally ill patient is the foundation of clinical care because it continues when cure is no longer possible. The nurse has a pivotal and privileged role in supporting patients, their families and friends through an extremely difficult physical and emotional experience (Kissane & Yates, 2003). The provision of palliative and supportive care for patients with advanced disease and their carers can be both demanding and complicated. It is important to recognise that this is a very stressful role for healthcare professionals and in order to care for these vulnerable groups effectively they need to identify their own needs and seek support appropriately.

REFERENCES

Ahlberg K, Ekman T, Gaston-Johansson F, Mock V (2003) Assessment and management of cancer-related fatigue in adults. *Lancet* **362**: 640–643.

Anderson K, Anderson LE, Glanze WD (eds) (1994) *Mosby's Medical, Medical, Nursing And Allied Health Dictionary*, 4th edn. Mosby, USA.

Aranda S (2003) A framework for symptom assessment. In: *Palliative Care Nursing: A Guide to Practice* (eds M O'Connor, S Aranda), 2nd edn, pp. 89–98. Radcliffe Medical Press, Oxford.

Back I (2001) *Palliative Medicine Handbook*, 3rd edn. BPM Books, Cardiff.

Baines MJ (1997) Nausea, vomiting and intestinal obstruction. *BM J* **315**: 1148–1150.

Baines M (1998) The pathophysiology and management of malignant intestinal obstruction. In: *Oxford Textbook of Palliative Medicine* (eds D Doyle, GWC Hanks, & N Macdonald), pp. 311–315. Oxford University Press, Oxford.

Barraclough J (1997) ABC of palliative care: Depression, anxiety and confusion. *BMJ* **315**: 1365–1368.

Bruera E, MacDonald RN (1988) Nutrition in cancer patients: an update and review of our experience. *J Pain Symptom Manage*, **3**(30): 133–140.

Dickman A, Schneider J, Varga J (2005) *The Syringe Driver Continuous Subcutaneous Infusions in Palliative Care*, 2nd edn. Oxford University Press, Oxford.

Flynn E, Quinn K (2003) Confusion and terminal restlessness. In: *Palliative Care Nursing. A Guide to Practice* (eds M O'Connor & S Aranda) 2nd edn. pp. 215–228. Radcliffe Medical Press Ltd, Oxford.

Hawthorn J (1995) *Understanding and Management of Nausea and Vomiting*. Blackwell Publishing, Oxford.

Hill S (2006) Symptom management: A framework. In: *Stepping into Palliative Care 2, Care and Practice* (ed. J Cooper). Radcliffe Publishing Ltd, Oxford.

Kaye P (1992) *A to Z of Hospice and Palliative Care*. EPL Publications, England.

Kaye P (2003) *A-Z Pocketbook of Symptom Control* 2nd edn. EPL Publications, UK.

Kissane D, Yates P (2003) Psychological and existential distress. In: *Palliative Care Nursing A Guide to Practice* (eds M O'Connor & S Aranda), 2nd edn. pp. 229–243. Radcliffe Medical Press, Oxford.

Lane I (2005) Managing cancer-related fatigue in palliative care. *Nurs Times* **101**(18): 38–41.

Lewis SJ, Heaton KW (1997) Stool form scale as a useful guide to intestinal transit time. *Scand J Gastroenterol* **32**(9): 920–924.

Martin J, Mehta DK (eds) (2007) *British National Formulary*. BMJ Publishing Group Ltd, London.

Meares CJ (2000) Nutritional issues in palliative care. *Seminars Oncol Nurs*, **16**(2): 135–145.

Millership R (2003) Nausea and vomiting. In: *Palliative Care Nursing: A Guide to Practice* (eds M O'Connor, & S Aranda) 2nd edn. pp. 173–185. Radcliffe Medical Press, Oxford.

Mitten T (2006) Introduction to pain management. In: *Stepping into Palliative Care* (ed J Cooper), 2nd edn. pp. 16–38. Radcliffe Publishing Ltd, Oxford.

Napp Pharmaceuticals Limited (2006). *MIMS Handbook of Pain Management*, 4th edn. Medical Imprints, London.

National Council for Palliative Care (2006). *Introductory Guide to End of Life Care in the Home*. National Council for Palliative Care, London.

O'Connor M (2003) Nutrition and hydration. In: *Palliative Care Nursing A Guide to Practice* (eds M O'Connor & S Aranda) 2nd edn. pp.187–197. Radcliffe Medical Press, Oxford.

Paz S, Seymour J (2004) Pain: Theories, Evaluation and Management. In: *Palliative Care Nursing: Principles and Evidence for Practice* (eds S Payne, J Seymour & C Ingleton). Open University Press, Oxford.

Porock D (2003) Fatigue. In: *Palliative Care Nursing A Guide to Practice* (eds M O'Connor & S Aranda), 2nd edn. pp. 137–152. Radcliffe Medical Press Ltd, Oxford.

Regnard C, Kindlen M, Dryden S, Mannix K, Alport S (2004) Nausea and vomiting. In: *Helping the Patient with Advanced Disease – a Workbook* (ed. C. Regnard) pp. 65–68. Radcliffe Medical Press Ltd, Oxford.

Ross DD, Alexander CS (2001) Management of common symptoms in terminally ill patients: Part 1. *Am Fam Physician*, 907–814.

Schofield P, Smith P, Aveyard B, Black C (2007) Complementary therapies for pain management in palliative care. *J Commun Nursing* **21**(8): 10–16.

Skalla K, Lacasse C (1992) Patient education for fatigue. *Oncol Nursing Forum* **19**: 1537–1541.

Stannard C, Booth S (2004) *Pain*. Churchill Livingstone, Edinburgh.

Thompson I (2004) The management of nausea and vomiting in palliative care. *Nurs Standard* **19**(8): 46–54.

Thornes A, Garrard E (2003) Ethical issues in care of the dying. In: *Care of the dying. A Pathway to Excellence* (eds J Ellershaw, & S Wilkinson). pp. 62–73. Oxford University Press, New York.

Twycross R (1997) *Symptom Management in Advanced Cancer*, 2nd edn. Radcliffe Medical Press Ltd, Oxford.

Twycross R (1999) Guidelines for the management of nausea and vomiting. *Palliative Care Today* **vii**(iv): 32–34.

Twycross R, Wilcock A (2001) *Symptom Management in Advanced Cancer*, 3rd edn. Radcliffe Medical Press Ltd, Oxford.

Watson M, Lucas C, Hoy A (2006) *Adult Palliative Care Guidance* 2nd edn. Surrey West Sussex Hampshire (SWSH) Mount Vernon and Sussex Cancer Networks and Northern Ireland Palliative Medicine Group, South West London.

West Midlands Palliative Care Physicians (2007) *Palliative Care Guidelines for the Use of Drugs in Symptom Control*, 4th edn. Independent Publisher, West Midlands.

Do Not Attempt Resuscitation Decisions

3

Elaine Walton and Philip Jevon

INTRODUCTION

The main purpose of medical treatment is to benefit the patient by restoring or maintaining health as far as possible, maximising benefit and minimising harm; if treatment is not beneficial, or if an adult competent patient refuses treatment, the purpose of medical treatment cannot be realised and the justification for providing it is removed (British Medical Association (BMA), Resuscitation Council UK & Royal College of Nursing (RCN), 2007).

Cardiopulmonary resuscitation (CPR) is a form of treatment that can in theory be undertaken in any patient when cardiac or respiratory function ceases. However, as failure of these functions is inevitable when a patient dies, it is important to identify patients for whom cardiopulmonary arrest represents a terminal event in their illness and in whom CPR is not beneficial and therefore inappropriate. When CPR is inappropriate, or is indeed against the wishes of a patient who is mentally competent, a 'do not attempt resuscitation' (DNAR) decision should be considered.

Decisions relating to cardiopulmonary resuscitation, the updated joint statement from the BMA, Resuscitation Council (UK) and the RCN (2007), outlines the ethical and legal standards for planning patient care and decision-making in relation to CPR.

The nurse has a professional responsibility to ensure that the patient's best interests and well-being are always promoted and safeguarded (Nursing and Midwifery Council (NMC), 2008).

The aim of this chapter is to understand the principles of DNAR decisions.

LEARNING OUTCOMES

At the end of the chapter, the reader will be able to:

❏ Discuss the historical background to DNAR decisions.
❏ Discuss the importance of DNAR decisions.
❏ List the key messages in *Decisions relating to cardiopulmonary resuscitation*.
❏ Provide an overview of the DNAR decision-making process.
❏ Outline factors underpinning DNAR decisions.
❏ Discuss the documentation of DNAR decisions.
❏ Outline DNAR written information requirements for patients and relatives.

HISTORICAL BACKGROUND TO DNAR DECISIONS

Historically, issuing a DNAR decision was considered part of the doctor's 'therapeutic prerogative', and often not formally registered in the patient's records, but 'understood' or 'indicated' by secret markings in records or on the bed (Holm & Jorgenson, 2001). Such practices may still exist where medical litigation is uncommon and there are no formal guidelines or policies.

In some situations, discussion and consultation about DNAR decisions had been carried out by staff least experienced or equipped to undertake such sensitive tasks (BMA, 1999). In addition, poor communication and documentation in respect of DNAR decisions could result in CPR being carried out or withheld inappropriately.

Nurses often left DNAR decisions to their medical colleagues; it is perhaps deemed easier to follow medical orders than be the patient's advocate and take on board their values and wishes.

Concerns regarding DNAR decisions

Concerns have been raised regarding DNAR decisions. In 1991, following a case brought to the attention of the Health Service Commissioner regarding a very junior doctor making a DNAR decision, the then Chief Medical Officer wrote to all consultants in England, reiterating their responsibility for ensuring a resuscitation policy was in place and understood by all staff who may be involved, particularly junior medical staff (Chief Medical Officer, 1991).

The much-publicised case of Kathryn Knight in 2000, a 67-year-old lady with an inoperable gastric carcinoma, highlighted concerns regarding DNAR decisions (Baker, 2000). She had been admitted to hospital with septicaemia (probably a complication of chemotherapy). A junior doctor, who had never seen or consulted Ms Knight, documented in her notes 'in view of the diagnosis, in the event of a cardiac arrest it would be inappropriate to resuscitate'. To make matters worse, Ms Knight was not informed of the decision. She only found out by chance about it during an outpatient department consultation.

In April 2000, Age Concern issued a press release stating that some doctors were ignoring national guidelines on the resuscitation of older people and that older people had found 'not for resuscitation' recorded in their medical notes without their agreement or knowledge (Luttrell, 2001). This lead Professor Shah Ebrahim to publish an editorial in the *British Medical Journal* stating that doctors regularly issue 'do not resuscitate' orders for patients without their knowledge; he claimed that black people, alcohol misusers, non-English speakers and those with HIV are more likely to get a DNAR order, suggesting that prejudice is influencing medical decisions (Ebrahim, 2000).

This combination of events was followed by intense media interest and concern regarding how DNAR decisions were being made. Such was the level of concern that the National Health Service (NHS) Executive issued a health service circular to all NHS Trust Chief Executives in September 2000 stipulating that appropriate resuscitation policies should be in place which respected patients' rights, were understood by all relevant staff and were subject to appropriate audit and monitoring (NHS Executive, 2000).

Media interest in DNAR decisions remains. The *Daily Mail* in its report 'Hospital gave order to let our mother die, say sisters', states that 'an elderly woman was left to die in hospital after an order not to resuscitate her was issued without her family's knowledge' (*Daily Mail*, 2008).

BMA, Resuscitation Council (UK) and the RCN guidelines

To improve DNAR decision-making, the BMA, Resuscitation Council (UK) and the RCN have produced guidelines on how and when DNAR decisions should be considered. First published in 1993 (BMA, 1993), these guidelines have been subsequently revised and updated (BMA, 1999, 2001); the latest guidelines, *Decisions relating to cardiopulmonary resuscitation*, were published in October 2007 and take into account the Mental Capacity Act 2005 (BMA *et al.*, 2007).

The guidelines provide a framework to:

- Support decisions relating to CPR.
- Ensure effective communication.
- Provide the general principles that allow for CPR policies to be tailored to local circumstances.

(BMA *et al.*, 2007)

Local policies may then provide further, more detailed, guidance, for example related to information about individual responsibilities (BMA *et al.*, 2007).

All healthcare organisations/providers that have to make decisions regarding resuscitation, e.g. hospitals, GP surgeries, care homes and ambulance services, should have a resuscitation policy which includes DNAR decisions (BMA *et al.*, 2007); this policy should be readily available and understood by all relevant staff (NHS Executive, 2000).

IMPORTANCE OF DNAR DECISIONS

Kouwenhoven and his colleagues first described closed-chest cardiac massage in the 1960s (Kouwenhoven *et al.*, 1960). They commented, 'anyone, anywhere, can now initiate cardiac resuscitative procedures. All that is needed are two hands'.

However, although modern resuscitation techniques have resulted in the successful resuscitation of many patients, they unfortunately have also made it possible to bring 'dead' patients back to life, prolong the process of dying and deny patients dignified and peaceful deaths with their close family present. 'You can treat and must not kill, but do not try to bring a dead soul back to life' (Pinder, 5th century BC cited in Negovsky, 1993).

It has been shown that, following a cardiac arrest in hospital, 50% of patients do not survive the CPR attempt (Tunstall-Pedoe *et al.*, 1992; Holland *et al.*, 1998), while less than 20% survive to discharge (Tunstall-Pedoe *et al.*, 1992). In 25% of CPR attempts, the process of dying is merely being prolonged (Snowden *et al.*, 1984). Resuscitation attempts are unsuccessful in 70–95% of cases and death is ultimately inevitable (Baskett *et al.*, 2005).

A valid DNAR decision is therefore important to prevent unnecessary CPR.

KEY MESSAGES IN *DECISIONS RELATING TO CARDIOPULMONARY RESUSCITATION*

The key messages in *Decisions relating to cardiopulmonary resuscitation* are:

- Decisions about CPR should be made following an individual assessment of the patient's case.
- Advance care planning, which should include decisions relating to CPR, is an important aspect of the sound clinical management of patients at risk of cardiorespiratory arrest.
- Communication and the provision of information are essential parts of effective quality care.
- Discussion about CPR is not necessary if the patient is unlikely to suffer a cardiorespiratory arrest.
- If no explicit decision has been made in advance, there should be initial presumption in favour of CPR.
- If CPR would not re-start the heart and breathing, it should not be attempted.
- If the anticipated benefits of performing CPR could be outweighed by the burdens, the patient's informed views are of paramount importance; if the patient lacks capacity, those close to him or her should be included in discussions to try to establish his or her wishes, feelings, beliefs and values.
- If a patient with capacity refuses CPR, or a patient lacking capacity has a valid and applicable advance decision refusing CPR, his or her wishes should be respected.
- A DNAR order decision does not override clinical judgement in the rare event when the cardiac arrest has a reversible cause that does not match the circumstances envisaged.

- A DNAR decision applies only to CPR, not to any other aspects of treatment.

(BMA *et al.*, 2007)

OVERVIEW OF THE DNAR DECISION-MAKING PROCESS

The flowchart in Figure 3.1 provides an overview of the DNAR decision-making process. This provides clear guidance to procedures that should be followed when considering a DNAR decision.

FACTORS UNDERPINNING DNAR DECISIONS

Importance of advance care planning

The risk of cardiopulmonary arrest is low in the majority of patients who receive health care in the hospital and community setting; there is no ethical or legal requirement to discuss every possible eventuality with the patient. If the risk of cardiopulmonary arrest is considered to be low, then it is not necessary to initiate discussion about CPR (BMA *et al.*, 2007).

However, there are patients who will be identified at risk of cardiopulmonary arrest, e.g. those with an incurable underlying condition, e.g. cancer, a severe acute illness, e.g. stroke, or at the end-of-life stage, for whom it would be desirable to make decisions regarding CPR (BMA *et al.*, 2007). Appropriate advanced care planning should be considered an essential component in good clinical practice.

Justification for treatment

The aim of health care is to benefit the patient by restoring/maintaining health, maximising benefit and minimising harm; treatment can no longer be justified if it fails or ceases to be beneficial, or if an adult patient with capacity refuses treatment (BMA *et al.*, 2007).

Although prolonging life can be beneficial, it is not appropriate to do so at all costs with no regard to quality of life or to the potential burdens the treatment ('successful CPR') will bring to the patient; the decision to undertake CPR should be based on the balance of burdens, risks and benefits to the patient (BMA *et al.*, 2007).

Decision-making framework

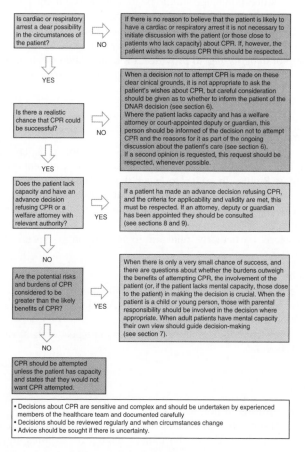

Is cardiac or respiratory arrest a dear possibility in the circumstances of the patient? **NO**

If there is no reason to believe that the patient is likely to have a cardiac or respiratory arrest it is not necessary to initiate discussion with the patient (or those close to patients who lack capacity) about CPR. If, however, the patient wishes to discuss CPR this should be respected.

YES

Is there a realistic chance that CPR could be successful? **NO**

When a decision not to attempt CPR is made on these clear clinical grounds, it is not appropriate to ask the patient's wishes about CPR, but careful consideration should be given as to whether to inform the patient of the DNAR decision (see section 6).
Where the patient lacks capacity and has a welfare attorney or court-appointed deputy or guardian, this person should be informed of the decision not to attempt CPR and the reasons for it as part of the ongoing discussion about the patient's care (see section 6).
If a second opinion is requested, this request should be respected, whenever possible.

YES

Does the patient lack capacity and have an advance decision refusing CPR or a welfare attorney with relevant authority? **YES**

If a patient ha made an advance decision refusing CPR, and the criteria for applicability and validity are met, this must be respected. If an attorney, deputy or guardian has been appointed they should be consulted (see sections 8 and 9).

NO

Are the potential risks and burdens of CPR considered to be greater than the likely benefits of CPR? **YES**

When there is only a very small chance of success, and there are questions about whether the burdens outweigh the benefits of attempting CPR, the involvement of the patient (or, if the patient lacks mental capacity, those dose to the patient) in making the decision is crucial. When the patient is a child or young person, those with parental responsibility should be involved in the decision where appropriate. When adult patients have mental capacity their own view should guide decision-making (see section 7).

NO

CPR should be attempted unless the patient has capacity and states that they would not want CPR attempted.

- Decisions about CPR are sensitive and complex and should be undertaken by experienced members of the healthcare team and documented carefully
- Decisions should be reviewed regularly and when circumstances change
- Advice should be sought if there is uncertainty.

Decisions relating to cardiopulmonary resuscitation

Fig 3.1 Decision-making framework for Do Not Attempt Resuscitation

Non-discrimination

Any CPR decision made should be individualised to the patient's particular circumstances and should not be influenced by age, disability or a healthcare professional's personal view of the patient's quality of life; a blanket policy that denies a particular group of patients, e.g. to provide CPR to all patients in a hospice would be considered unethical and probably unlawful (BMA *et al.*, 2007).

Human Rights Act 1998

The Human Rights Act 1998 incorporates into UK law the majority of rights set out in the European Convention on Human Rights. In order to meet their obligations under the Act, health professionals must be able to demonstrate that their decisions are compatible with the human rights identified in Articles of the Convention (Resuscitation Council UK, 2000). Provisions particularly relevant to DNAR orders include the right to:

- Life (Article 2).
- Be free from inhuman or degrading treatment (Article 3).
- Respect for privacy and family life (Article 8).
- Freedom of expression (Article 10).
- Be free from discriminatory practices in respect of these rights (Article 14).

(BMA *et al.*, 2007)

Presumptions in favour of CPR

In the absence of a valid DNAR decision, CPR should be commenced in the event of the patient having a cardiorespiratory arrest.

However, if CPR is inappropriate, e.g. a patient who is in the final stages of a terminal illness, where death is imminent and CPR would be unsuccessful, it should not be started even in the absence of a DNAR decision; a nurse who makes a considered decision not to start CPR should be supported by colleagues and her employer (BMA *et al.*, 2007).

Mental Health Act 2005 and Adults with Incapacity Act 2000

The Mental Health Act 2005 (England and Wales) and the Adults with Incapacity Act 2000 (Scotland) provide guidance concerning proxy decision-makers and their role when the patient lacks decision-making capacity (lacks capacity). More detailed information can be found in Chapter 10.

Liverpool Care Pathway

The Liverpool Care Pathway (LCP) (see pp. 8–10), which is currently being implemented across the UK, provides a comprehensive evidence-based template for multidisciplinary care for last few days of life; Goal 3 of the initial assessment specifically reminds the clinician to consider and document the patient's CPR status (BMA *et al.*, 2007).

Who can make a DNAR decision?

The overall responsibility for making a DNAR decision rests with the most senior clinician in charge of the patient's care as defined by the local DNAR policy (it may be delegated to another competent person) (BMA *et al.*, 2007); in most situations this will be a registered medical practitioner but in some situations, such as in nurse-led palliative care services, a senior nurse with appropriate training may fulfil this role, subject to local discussion and agreement (BMA *et al.*, 2007).

A DNAR decision should ideally be agreed with other appropriate members of the healthcare team (BMA *et al.*, 2007); if there is genuine doubt or disagreement about whether CPR would be clinically appropriate, a further senior clinical opinion should be sought (BMA *et al.*, 2007).

The nurse must always act in such a manner as to promote and safeguard the interests and well-being of the patient and should recognise and respect the uniqueness and dignity of every patient (NMC, 2008). If the nurse is of the opinion that CPR is not appropriate for a patient, or is indeed aware that the patient does not wish to be resuscitated in the event of a cardiac arrest, then he or she should raise the issue with senior medical colleagues at the earliest opportunity. In some situations, as described earlier, the senior nurse will be making the DNAR decision (BMA *et al.*, 2007).

DNAR decision based on clinical decision

In some cases, a DNAR decision is made on clinical grounds, i.e. CPR will not be successful at restarting breathing and circulation. In these situations, it is not necessary or appropriate to ascertain the patient's wishes regarding CPR, unless the patient has expressed a specific wish to do so (BMA *et al.*, 2007). It is usual practice to inform relatives of the decision.

DNAR decision based on benefits and burdens

A DNAR decision based on balancing the benefits and burdens of CPR should take into account the:

- Likely clinical outcome and level of realistic recovery.
- Patient's own or ascertainable wishes, views, feelings, beliefs and values.
- Patient's human rights (see Human Rights Act 1998).
- Likelihood of the patient experiencing severe unmanageable pain or suffering.
- Level of the patient's awareness of his or her existence and surroundings.

(BMA *et al.*, 2007)

Should the patient be consulted?

The rights of the patient are central to decision-making on resuscitation. Patients have as much right to be involved in DNAR decisions as they do with other decisions about their care and treatment (Department of Health (DH), 2000). In fact, approximately 90% of patients would prefer to discuss the issue of CPR and there are often inconsistencies between what the patient wants and what the medical staff think the patient wants (Broekman, 1998). When a DNAR decision is based on considerations related to established benefits and burdens, the views of the patient should be sought (BMA *et al.*, 2007).

However, when a DNAR decision is made on clinical grounds, i.e. CPR will not be successful at restarting breathing and circulation, it is unnecessary and inappropriate to explore the patient's wishes regarding CPR, unless a specific wish to do so is expressed by the patient (BMA *et al.*, 2007).

Patient with capacity

If a patient with capacity (mental power) is at risk of cardiac or respiratory arrest, and the healthcare team is doubtful whether the benefits of undertaking CPR outweigh the burdens and whether the predicted post-successful recovery will be acceptable for the patient, sensitive exploration of the patient's wishes, feelings, beliefs and values should be sought (BMA *et al.*, 2007). Any discussions with the patient should be accurately documented.

Clinicians who discuss or communicate DNAR decisions with patients should:

- Provide patients with as much information as they wish.
- Provide information in such a manner and format that patients can understand it (an interpreter may be required).
- Answer questions as honestly as possible.
- Explain the aims of treatment.

(BMA *et al.*, 2007)

If a patient does not accept a DNAR decision which has been made on clinical grounds, then careful explanation of reasons for the decision is required; if requested, a second opinion should be arranged wherever possible (the same procedure applies to relatives should they disagree with a DNAR decision (BMA *et al.*, 2007).

Patient who lacks capacity

If a patient who lacks capacity is at risk of cardiac or respiratory arrest, and the healthcare team is doubtful whether the benefits of undertaking CPR will outweigh the burdens, discussions should take place within the healthcare team about a DNAR decision (BMA *et al.*, 2007). The patient's best interests must be central to the decision-making process.

Relatives

Those close to the patient should be consulted; this is considered good practice and is probably a requirement of the Human Rights

Act 1998 (Article 8 – right to private and family life; Article 10 – right to impart and receive information) and the Mental Capacity Act (2005) (BMA *et al.*, 2007). It must be emphasised that those close to the patient have no legal authority in the decision-making process and that their role is purely to help the clinician in the decision-making process.

Lasting power of attorney

The Mental Capacity Act 2005 (England and Wales) allows adults who have capacity to make a lasting power of attorney (LPA), appointing someone to make decisions regarding their health care (welfare attorney), should they ever lack the capacity to make the decisions themselves (BMA *et al.*, 2007). An attorney is a person, especially a lawyer, appointed to act for another in business or legal matters (*The Concise Oxford Dictionary*, 1998).

However, before relying on the authority of the welfare attorney, the healthcare team should be satisfied that:

- The patient lacks capacity to make a DNAR decision.
- A statement has been included in the LPA, stipulating that the welfare attorney can make decisions about life-prolonging treatment.
- The LPA has been registered with the Office of the Public Guardian.
- The decision made by the welfare attorney is in the best interests of the patient.

(BMA *et al.*, 2007)

If CPR is clinically inappropriate, the welfare attorney cannot demand that it be carried out. However, if CPR is likely to restart the heart and the DNAR decision will be based on the balance between benefits and burdens, the welfare attorney should be consulted regarding the patient's likely wishes; if there is a disagreement which cannot be resolved through discussion and a second clinical opinion, the court of protection may be asked to make a declaration (BMA *et al.*, 2007).

Mental capacity advocate

The Mental Capacity Act 2005 stipulates that an independent mental capacity advocate (IMCA) should be consulted regarding all decisions about serious medical treatment, where the patient lacks capacity and there is no one, e.g. relative or welfare attorney, who is able to speak on the patient's behalf. Where there is genuine doubt whether CPR would be successful or if a DNAR decision is being considered on the balance of benefits and burdens, an IMCA must be involved (BMA *et al.*, 2007). If a DNAR decision is being considered, but an IMCA is not available (e.g. at night or at a weekend), it should be discussed with the IMCA at the earliest opportunity (BMA *et al.*, 2007).

Advance decisions
An advance decision (formally referred to as advance directive or living will) is related to end-of-life treatment. It should be in writing, and as long as it is valid and applicable, should be followed and treatment not provided. It takes precedence over any view that anyone else may have about what is in the best interests of the person in question, even if the result is that the decision results in the person dying. Advance decisions are discussed in detail in Chapter 10.

When to ignore or suspend a DNAR decision
Occasionally, a patient with a DNAR decision may suffer a cardiac or respiratory arrest caused by a readily reversible cause, e.g. choking on a foreign body or anaphylaxis. In these rare situations, unless the patient has specifically refused intervention, it would be appropriate to initiate CPR (BMA *et al.*, 2007).

Similarly, it may be appropriate to suspend a DNAR decision if the patient is undertaking a procedure which carries a risk of a potentially reversible cardiac arrest, e.g. cardiac catheterisation (ventricular fibrillation) (BMA *et al.*, 2007).

DOCUMENTATION OF DNAR DECISIONS
Any discussions with the patient, relatives and healthcare team regarding DNAR decisions should be documented, signed and dated in the patient's health records. It should also be documented if patients have stated they do not wish to be involved in such discussions.

To avoid confusion, it is recommended to use the phrase 'Do Not Attempt Cardiopulmonary Resuscitation' when documenting a DNAR decision (BMA *et al.*, 2007). In addition, other pertinent information should be documented, following local guidelines, including:

- Date and time the decision was made.
- Who made the decision.
- Rationale.
- Discussions with patient, relatives and healthcare team.
- Review date/time.

DNAR decisions should be reviewed on a regular basis, which should be determined by the clinician in charge and will be influenced by the clinical circumstances of the patient. Local policies should include safeguards to ensure that a review occurs appropriately, and that the patient's ability to participate in the decision-making process might change depending on his or her clinical condition. However, it is generally not necessary to discuss the DNAR decision with the patient every time it is reviewed, unless the decision is changed (BMA, *et al.*, 2007).

Some healthcare establishments have devised DNAR forms to assist the clinician with making a DNAR decision (Figure 3.2). These have been seen to improve the clarity of the DNAR statement, particularly by whom, when it has been documented and reasons for the decision (Castle *et al.*, 2003; Diggory *et al.*, 2003, 2004; Cauchi *et al.*, 2004; Harris & Linnane, 2005). The Resuscitation Council UK is currently in the process of developing a model DNAR form that individual establishments might wish to adopt (www.resus.org.uk; accessed 7 January 2008). This is to assist healthcare staff with ensuring that all relevant aspects of the order are covered and also making it easier to recognise and use forms immediately.

INFORMATION FOR PATIENTS AND RELATIVES

The BMA's Ethics Department has issued a model patient leaflet *Decisions relating to cardiopulmonary resuscitation* (BMA, 2002). It provides patients with information to assist them in making decisions related to their treatment and may be useful to relatives, friends and carers. It states what CPR is and whether it is relevant to consider issues related to this, and how decisions are made about whether it should be attempted or not. This model

Walsall Hospitals NHS Trust

RESUSCITATION STATUS CHECK LIST (*ONLY TO BE USED WHEN A DNAR ORDER PLACED*)

On discharge please return **top copy** to Resuscitation Training Office (RTO), Education & Training Dept.
Bottom copy to remain in patient notes

(patient details - attach label)

Ward / Dept:
Admission date:
Discharge date:

1 Date/Time	2 Do Not Attempt Resus Order in Place (Y/N)	3 On Review, Patient for Resus (Y/N)	4 Discussed with patient (Y/N)	5 Discussed with others (relatives) (Y/N)	6 Decision made by (PRINT NAME)	7 Signature	8 Status	9 Review Date/Time
	Y							

JB-335586

WOEM44

Fig 3.2 A DNAR flowchart to assist the clinician with making a DNAR decision. Reproduced by kind permission of Walsall Hospitals NHS Trust

information leaflet can be amended to include local information and can be obtained from the BMA's website (www.bma.org.uk).

Such information should be readily available to all patients and people close to the patient, and written information about CPR policies should be included in the general literature provided to patients about healthcare organisations. A sample patient information leaflet is depicted in Figure 3.3. In addition, the DNAR policy should be readily available to those who might wish to consult it, including patients, relatives and carers (DH, 2000).

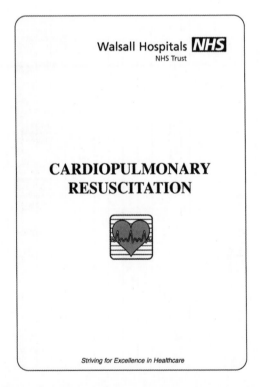

Fig 3.3 Cardiopulmonary resuscitation: a sample patient information leaflet. Reproduced by kind permission of Walsall Hopsitals NHS Trust

CONCLUSION

In this chapter, an overview to DNAR decisions has been provided. The historical background to DNAR decisions and their importance have been discussed. The key messages in *Decisions relating to cardiopulmonary resuscitation* have been listed and an overview of the DNAR decision-making process has been provided. The factors underpinning DNAR decisions have been highlighted, together with documentation issues and written information requirements for patients and relatives.

Further information

Medical Ethics Department
British Medical Association
BMA House
Tavistock Square
London WC1H 9JP
Tel 020 7383 6286

Resuscitation Council (UK)
5th Floor, Tavistock House North
Tavistock Square
London WC1H 9HR
Tel 020 7388 4678

Royal College of Nursing
20 Cavendish Square
London W1 OAB
Tel 020 7409 3333

REFERENCES

Baker J (2000) Doctors were told to just let me die. *Daily Express*, 14 April.

Baskett P, Steen P, Bossaert L (2005) European Resuscitation Council Guidelines for Resuscitation 2005 Section 8. The ethics of resuscitation and end-of-life decisions *Resuscitation* S171–S180.

British Medical Association (BMA) (1993) *Decisions Relating to Cardiopulmonary Resuscitation. A Joint Statement from the British Medical Association, the Resuscitation Council (UK) and the Royal College of Nursing.* BMA, London.

British Medical Association (BMA) (1999) *Decisions Relating to Cardiopulmonary Resuscitation. A Joint Statement from the British Medical Association, the Resuscitation Council (UK) and the Royal College of Nursing.* BMA, London.

British Medical Association (BMA) (2001) *Decisions Relating to Cardiopulmonary Resuscitation. A Joint Statement from the British Medical Association, the Resuscitation Council (UK) and the Royal College of Nursing.* BMA, London.

British Medical Association BMA (2002) *Decisions Relating to Cardiopulmonary Resuscation (model information leaflet).* BMA, London.

British Medical Association (BMA), Resuscitation Council UK & Royal College of Nursing (2007) *Decisions Relating to Cardiopulmonary Resuscitation. A Joint Statement from the British Medical Association, the Resuscitation Council UK and the Royal College of Nursing.* BMA, London.

Broekman B (1998) Discussing resuscitation with patients, why not? *Resuscitation* **37**(2): 062.

Castle N, Owen R, Kenwood G, Ineson N (2003) Pre-printed 'Do Not Attempt Resuscitation' forms improve documentation? *Resuscitation* **59**: 85–95.

Cauchi L, Vigus J, Diggory P (2004) Implementation of cardiopulmonary resuscitation in elderly care departments across: A survey of 13 hospitals shows wide variability in practice. *Resuscitation* **63**: 157–160.

Chief Medical Officer (1991) *(PL/CMO(91)22).* Department of Health, London.

Daily Mail (2008) Hospital gave order to let our mother die, say sisters. *Daily Mail*, 25 March, p. 32.y

Department of Health (DH) (2000) *Health Service Circular: Resuscitation Policy.* DH, London.

Diggory P, Cauchi L, Griffith D, *et al.* (2003) The influence of new guidelines on cardiopulmonary resuscitation (CPR) decisions. Five cycles of audit of a clerk proforma which included a resuscitation decision. *Resuscitation* **56**: 159–165.

Diggory P, Shire L, Griffith D, *et al.* (2004) Influence of guidelines on cardiopulmonary resuscitation (CPR) decisions: an audit of clerking proforma. *Clin Med* **4**: 424–426.

Ebrahim S (2000) Do not resuscitate decisions; flogging dead horses or a dignified death? *BMJ* **320**: 1155–1156.

Harris DG, Linnane SJ (2005) Making do not attempt resuscitation decisions: Do doctors follow the guidelines? *Hosp Med* **66**(1): 43–45.

Holland M, Hawkins J, Gill M, *et al.* (1998) One year prospective audit of outcome following cardiopulmonary resuscitation on an in-hospital patient population. *Resuscitation* **37**(2): 0103.

Holm S, Jorgenson EO (2001) Ethical issues in cardiopulmonary resuscitation. *Resuscitation* **50**: 135–139.

Kouwenhoven W, Jude J, Knickerbocker G (1960) Closed-chest cardiac massage. *JAMA* **173**: 1064–1067.

Luttrell S (2001) Decisions relating to cardiopulmonary resuscitation: Commentary 2: Some concerns. *J Med Ethics* **27**: 321–322.

NHS Executive (2000) *Resuscitation Policy (HSC 2000/028)*. Department of Health, London.

Negovsky VA (1993) Death, dying and revival: ethical aspects. *Resuscitation* **25**: 99–107.

Nursing and Midwifery Council (NMC) (2008) *The Code*. NMC, London.

Resuscitation Council (UK) (2000) *Advanced Life Support Provider Manual*. 4th Edn. Resuscitation Council (UK), London.

Snowden G, Baskett P, Robins D (1984) Factors associated with survival and eventual cerebral status following cardiac arrest. *Anaesthesia* **39**: 1.

Tunstall-Pedoe H, Bailey L, Chamberlain DA, Marsden AK, Ward ME, Zideman D, *et al.* (1992) Survey of 3765 cardiopulmonary resuscitations in British Hospitals. The BRESUS Study: methods and overall results. *BMJ* **304**: 1347–1351.

4 Ethical Issues

Fiona Foxall

INTRODUCTION

All nurses will inevitably encounter the death of a patient and in some cases ethical dilemmas will be raised, which may cause anxiety and confusion for those caring for the patient. Concerns relating to the possible use of futile treatment, which does not appear to be in the best interests of their patient; the withholding and withdrawal of active treatment; patients in a persistent vegetative state and the ethical issues this condition raises and the emotive concept of euthanasia may all seem difficult to interpret and apply in practice.

The aim of this chapter is to provide an overview to the ethical issues.

LEARNING OUTCOMES

At the end of the chapter, the reader will be able to:

❏ Outline the major ethical theories and principles.
❏ Discuss the concept of medical futility.
❏ Outline the principles of acting in the best interests of the patient.
❏ Discuss the ethics of withholding and withdrawing active treatment.
❏ Discuss the ethical concerns surrounding persistent vegetative state.
❏ Discuss the ethical concepts of euthanasia.

ETHICAL THEORIES AND PRINCIPLES

There are two major ethical theories that guide healthcare practice: deontology (duty-based theory), the basic tenet of which is, 'I must always carry out my duty', and utilitarianism (consequence-based theory), which asserts that an action is right if it produces the greatest benefit for the greatest number of people.

In addition, there are four guiding ethical principles that should be used in any decision-making process:

- *Non-maleficence* – (primum non nocere) first and above all – do no harm.
- *Beneficence* – do good, promote good, remove evil or harm.
- *Respect for autonomy* – taking into account and acting on the patient's wishes.
- *Justice* – fairness, entitlement or right.

(Beauchamp & Childress, 2001)

These theories and principles can aid decision-making by asking six simple questions:

- What is my duty in this particular circumstance?
- By carrying out my duty, will my actions produce the best available consequences for all concerned?
- Will my actions harm anyone, particularly the patient?
- Am I going to do or promote good for those concerned?
- Am I respecting the patient's wishes?
- Are my actions fair to all concerned?

Although this may over-simplify the decision-making process, it does provide a helpful ethical guide. The Code of Professional Conduct for Nurses, Midwives and Health Visitors (Nursing and Midwifery Council (NMC), 2002) takes these issues into account; therefore working within the confines of this code will ensure that you act not only within the law but also in a professional and ethical manner.

MEDICAL FUTILITY

The concept of medical futility refers to interventions that are unlikely to produce any significant benefit for the patient. This can be either in terms of the likelihood that an intervention will benefit the patient or if there is any benefit, in the quality of that benefit. A treatment that merely produces a physiological effect on a patient's body does not necessarily confer any benefit that the patient can appreciate. The question is, 'Does the intervention have any reasonable prospect of helping the patient?' (Jecker, 2000).

Healthcare professionals have no obligation to offer treatments or procedures that do not benefit patients. Futile treatments are ill-advised because they often increase the patient's pain and discomfort in the last days and weeks of life and because they could expend finite medical resources (Jecker, 2000).

Futility arises when there is no reasonable hope of recovery and speculative therapy attempts are made, which may result in greater harm to the patient than would have been the case had the therapy not been attempted. For example, cardiopulmonary resuscitation (CPR) has the ability to reverse premature death; it can also prolong terminal illness, increase discomfort and consume enormous resources (Ewanchuck & Brindley, 2006). Only 10–20% of all those in whom CPR is attempted in acute general hospitals will live i.e., survive and be discharged from hospital (Bowker & Stewart, 1999). It is therefore clear that CPR is often futile and, where appropriate, the healthcare team should consider a 'Do Not Attempt Resuscitation' (DNAR) order (BMA *et al.*, 2007).

The following two scenarios aid the consideration of the concept of medical futility.

Scenario 4.1

Sally is a 28-year-old woman who has been involved in a road traffic accident in which she sustained a serious head injury culminating in an intraventricular haemorrhage. Whilst in the emergency department she suffered a cardiac arrest. The advanced life support measures restored her circulation but she required artificial ventilation as she was making no respiratory effort. She was admitted to the intensive care unit and was ventilated for three days. On the third day, Sally suffered a further cardiac arrest and despite all attempts at CPR, no cardiac function could be maintained.

• Is artificial ventilation now futile?

In this case, it is quite clear that any further treatment would be considered futile as the patient is unquestionably dead, although she is still on a ventilator but she can no longer be harmed by the cessation of treatment (Beauchamp & Childress, 2001). This may seem obvious but is a very important point because healthcare professionals do not only make decisions about the futility of a treatment once the patient has died.

Scenario 4.2

Arthur is 76 years old and was diagnosed with prostate cancer two weeks ago. The disease is in the early stages and surgery is planned for the near future, which is expected to be success-ful. He lives in a residential home for the elderly since his family felt he could not cope living alone because he suffers with dementia. He is frequently confused and does not recognise his family during these periods of confusion. However, he also has periods of lucidity, although these periods are reducing in time and frequency but whilst lucid he is chatty and happy.

Arthur has been admitted to an acute medical ward as he has developed pneumonia and requires antibiotics.

• Should antibiotics be prescribed for Arthur?

Arthur's quality of life may seem to be low, but it is not unac-ceptably so and in this situation, antibiotic therapy would stand a reasonable chance of successfully treating the patient's pneu-monia. Unless Arthur has a written advance directive or has expressed an objection to such treatment during lucid phases, there are no grounds for calling antibiotic therapy futile in this case. The situation may seem undesirable; however, undesirable is quite different from futile and healthcare professionals must be careful in their decision-making to accurately assess specific situations so that futility is not interpreted inaccurately by making value judgements.

ACTING IN THE BEST INTERESTS OF THE PATIENT

Acting in the best interests of the patient is probably one of the most fundamental principles of health care. It is indeed the very essence of ethical care. In this context, the word 'best' relates to what is good for the patient, that is what will undoubtedly be of benefit. 'Interests' of course also relate to what will be of benefit to the patient. The benefit of treatment must be viewed in terms of net benefit, that is what will be in the best interests of the patient, all things considered (Devettere, 2000).

To explore the concept of acting in the best interests of the patient, consider the following scenarios.

Scenario 4.3

Harry is a 79-year-old man who has cancer of the bowel. He has previously undergone major surgery to remove a tumour and he has been treated with both chemotherapy and radiotherapy, to no avail. He now has metastatic disease, which is untreatable; he is very frail and will imminently die.

He also has a very painful ingrowing toenail, which could be easily treated by minor surgery, although it would be very painful in the post-operative period. The operation would provide some benefit, in that the pain in his toe would ultimately be reduced.

- Even though it will provide some benefit, would the surgery be in his best interests, all things considered?

Scenario 4.4

Hugh is a 79-year-old man who has advanced motor neurone disease. He has had all possible treatments and palliation but is now in a great deal of pain, which is difficult to control; he is very frail and will imminently die.

He has now developed pneumonia and requires antibiotics if he is to survive. Clearly, antibiotics would be of some benefit as they could halt the progress of the pneumonia.

- Even though antibiotics will provide some benefit, would the therapy be in his best interests, all things considered?

In considering these two scenarios, the decision about whether or not to apply the proposed treatments would be made in light of any benefit the patients would derive from the treatment. Clearly, there is some benefit from both courses of action outlined because the specific conditions for which the treatment would be applied would be improved.

However, in view of Harry's overwhelming malignant disease, the proposed surgery for his ingrowing toenail would be too burdensome and therefore not of overall benefit and thus, not in his best interests, all things considered (Devettere, 2000).

With regard to treating Hugh's pneumonia, antibiotics may indeed benefit him with regard to this infection. However, it would also possibly prolong his life or, rather, prolong his dying, which would not be of benefit overall and withholding the treatment would therefore reduce this burden.

The principle of beneficence is a moral obligation to act to benefit others or to act in the best interests of others. In healthcare, this may seem obvious as an obligation, but there is a risk that nurses may think that they know what is best for the patient. In our wish to do good for patients, we can override their autonomy and step beyond the boundary of beneficence into paternalism, i.e. the overriding of one person's preferences by another person, and possibly inflict harm.

Autonomy addresses personal freedom and self-determination – the right to choose what happens to one's own person (within social and legal constraints). The legal doctrine of informed consent is a direct reflection of this principle. Autonomy involves healthcare deliverers' respect for patients' rights to make decisions affecting care and treatment, even if the healthcare deliverers do not agree with the decisions made (Wacker Guido, 2006).

All competent patients have the right to decide what happens to their body, and their autonomous choices must be consulted whenever possible as the basis of any decision. Patients are competent to make a decision if they have the capacity to understand the material information, to make a judgement about the information in light of their values, to intend a certain outcome, and to communicate freely their wishes to caregivers (Beauchamp & Childress, 2001). Patients have fundamental legal and ethical rights in determining what happens to their own bodies (Department of Health (DH), 2001).

The legal and moral duty of care that is owed to vulnerable clients by those entrusted with their care is of vital importance and must not be overlooked (Fletcher & Buka, 1999). The Mental Capacity Act 2005 for England and Wales gained Royal Assent on 7 April 2007, and was implemented through stages during 2007 (Department for Constitutional Affairs 2007). The purpose of the Mental Capacity Act 2005 is to provide a legal framework to protect vulnerable people who may be assessed as being unable to make informed decisions regarding their own life and choices. The Act provides guidance on the decision-making process where decisions are being made on behalf of those who lack capacity.

Advance directives (also referred to as living wills, advance statements or advance refusals) are rooted in respect for autonomy, which is one of the foremost ethical principles (Beauchamp & Childress, 2001). Western society places great importance on a person's right to self-determination even when he or she is unable to participate in decision-making because of incompetence (De Wolf Bosek & Savage, 2007). As competent adults, patients have a right to refuse medical treatment; an advance directive is a way of prolonging autonomy. However, an advance directive cannot request treatment that is not in the best interests of the patient.

Advance directives are usually written directives from competent individuals to healthcare professionals regarding treatment that should be provided or forgone in specific circumstances, during periods of incompetence (Beauchamp & Childress, 2001). However, an advance directive does not have to be written to be valid. If a patient makes a verbal advance statement that they do not wish to have a particular form of treatment should they become incapacitated, this must be respected.

The trigger for using an advance directive is typically the occurrence of an acute clinical event in a patient with an enduring or degenerative condition that has already compromised quality of life as judged by the patient whilst competent, and does not wish his or her life to be protracted by artificial means.

The ethical principle of non-maleficence, the obligation not to inflict harm intentionally, is important here. Many treatments and procedures in health care cause harmful side-effects but the interventions save or improve quality of life overall. However, there are times when a patient's quality of life is so poor or the intervention would prove so burdensome that it is more appropriate to withhold or withdraw it, as the balance of harm over benefit is too great. The major considerations in end-of-life decision-making are the degree of harm being caused by interventions, whether that harm outweighs any benefits and indeed, whether death would be a harm in the circumstances.

THE ETHICS OF WITHDRAWAL OF ACTIVE TREATMENT

Few decisions are more momentous than those to withhold or withdraw a medical procedure that sustains life (Beauchamp & Childress, 2001). Difficulties may arise when caring for patients at the end of their lives who are unable to make decisions about continuation of treatment. Ethical dilemmas arise when there is a perceived conflicting duty to the patient, such as a conflict between the duty to preserve life and a duty to act in the patient's best interests, or when an ethical principle, such as respect for autonomy, conflicts with the duty not to harm. A number of ethical doctrines are relevant when considering the withdrawal of treatment and end-of-life decisions.

Sanctity of life doctrine

According to this doctrine, all human life has worth and therefore it is wrong to end a person's life, directly or indirectly, however poor the quality of that life (Glover, 1977). In health care this means preserving life at all costs but clearly, quality of life is hugely important to the majority of people. It is, however, very difficult to objectively assess the quality of a patient's life when you are not living that life. However, there may be circumstances where a patient's quality of life is deemed so poor, it is considered to be a life not worth living and therefore should not be maintained even if it is possible to do so.

Acts and omissions doctrine

This doctrine highlights the distinction between killing and letting die. There is a moral distinction between taking action to bring about a person's death and refraining from an action that might save or preserve a person's life (Rachels, 1975). For example, it is morally wrong to push someone who cannot swim into deep water; however, there is no moral duty to dive into a river to save someone who is drowning. In the context of health care, this would mean it is wrong to give a lethal injection to end a patient's life, but treatments that could sustain life can be withdrawn when they are no longer of benefit and, therefore, it is not in the best interests of the patient to continue. Withholding and withdrawing treatment are both considered omissions to act.

Doctrine of double effect

This doctrine asserts that there is a moral distinction between carrying out an action to bring about a person's death and carrying out an action that provides some benefit but as a result, the death of the person is a foreseen but unintended consequence (Beauchamp & Childress, 2001), for example giving high dosages of drugs to relieve pain (beneficial action), which will, however, shorten life (unintended consequence). The intention is to relieve pain but the death of the person is unintended although foreseeable.

End-of-life care must primarily be directed at providing symptom and pain management to patients for whom curative medicine is no longer an option. When further interventions are inappropriate, health professionals should provide comfort and the highest possible quality of life for as long as life remains: dictated by the concepts of beneficence and justice. The focus of end-of-life care should not be on death but on ensuring that the life that remains is as comfortable as possible.

In considering the appropriateness of care, sanctity versus quality of life issues need to be taken into account. The acts and omissions doctrine and the doctrine of double effect can be very useful in aiding the healthcare deliverer in determining treatment and care options.

For example, the question of whether a patient's life is not worth living because his or her quality of life is so poor, as determined by the patient and/or significant others, together with the healthcare team, can aid the decision of whether or not to withhold or withdraw particular treatments. Omitting to act is justifiable if the action is of no benefit to the patient. Increasing drug dosages to maintain a pain-free state for the patient is acceptable even if that action brings about death more swiftly because death is the unintended consequence of the beneficent act of killing pain.

The doctrine of double effect is important here, together with the principle of beneficence. The question that arises here is, 'is death a harm in this circumstance?'. If the answer is that the life is too burdensome for the patient, then it could be considered a life not worth living and death would not be a harm, but indeed a release from pain and therefore burden. The best person to determine the answer to this question is the patient. Pain reduces quality of life, therefore if pain is alleviated, the burden to the patient is reduced and quality of life improves even if that life is shorter as a result of treatments given.

It is justifiable to discontinue life-sustaining treatments if:

- Patients have the ability to make decisions, fully understand the consequences of their decisions and state they no longer want treatment.
- The treatment no longer offers benefit to the patients.

(Braddock, 1999)

Although many healthcare professionals feel it is more acceptable not to start a treatment than to withdraw it, there is actually no ethical distinction between withholding and withdrawing treatment (Braddock, 1999; Beauchamp & Childress, 2001).

PERSISTENT VEGETATIVE STATE
The persistent vegetative state (PVS) presents particular ethical concerns because the condition is so extreme in nature. It results in irreparable destruction to the brain cortex and, although patients appear to be in a state of wakefulness and reflex responses may remain, it is widely accepted that patients are unconscious (British Medical Association (BMA), 1996).

The patient in PVS can breathe spontaneously, has an independent heartbeat, and normal digestive, renal and other autonomic physiological functions. However, sight, hearing, taste, smell and communication in any form are totally absent; spontaneous movement is limited or absent; the patient is rendered insentient. No emotion can be expressed, as there is loss of all cognitive function and, as a result, such patients are incapable of suffering mental distress or physical pain. Although there have been some reports of recovery from PVS, the BMA (1996) maintains that this would indicate an original misdiagnosis.

The BMA recommends that decisions to withdraw treatment should only be considered when the patient has been insentient for 12 months. If there is any doubt about the reversibility of the condition, decisions about possible withdrawal of treatment must be deferred (BMA, 1996).

It is good medical practice to provide artificial nutrition and hydration to sustain any patient whose prognosis is uncertain. Medical treatments, including artificial nutrition and hydration, may be withdrawn at a later stage, after legal review of the case, if they are considered futile (BMA, 1996).

Consider the following two scenarios to determine the appropriate action to be taken for a patient in PVS.

Scenario 4.5

Janet is a 43-year-old lady who lost her footing and fell down a flight of stairs in a restaurant. She hit the top of her head on a fire extinguisher at the bottom of the staircase. She was admitted via the emergency department to the intensive care unit and then to the neurology ward and has been in hospital for six weeks. She has some reflex responses although gag and swallow reflexes are absent. She does not respond to commands although she opens her eyes spontaneously and appears occasionally to be awake.

The medical staff caring for her feel certain that she is in a PVS. She is currently receiving nutrition via a nasogastric tube but it is felt a percutaneous endoscopic gastrostomy (PEG) tube feed would now be more appropriate because of the long-term nature of her condition, which will involve a surgical procedure.

- Should the procedure be carried out?
- Should the feed be withdrawn?

Decisions to withdraw treatment should only be considered when Janet has been insentient for 12 months. Therefore, at this stage, there can be no certain diagnosis made. Hence, any decisions about possible withdrawal of treatment must be deferred and the provision of artificial nutrition and hydration to sustain Janet should continue until she has been in the same condition for 12 months, when her treatment can be reviewed and possibly be withdrawn, after a legal review of her case.

Scenario 4.6

Jenny is an 18-year-old girl who was involved in a road traffic accident in which she sustained a severe head injury and a crush injury to the chest. As a result, she has been in a PVS for almost two years. She has some reflex responses although gag and swallow reflexes are absent. She does not respond to commands although she opens her eyes spontaneously and appears occasionally to be awake.

She is fed via a PEG tube as she has no swallow reflex. Her parents and the healthcare professionals caring for her all feel she has a life of no quality and is therefore a life not worth living. The only way to end her life would be to cease the feed and allow her to die from malnutrition and dehydration.

- What should be done in this circumstance?

The legal position regarding cases such as Jenny's was clarified in England and Wales by the House of Lords in the Bland case (*Airedale NHS Trust v Bland* [1993], AC 789). Anthony Bland suffered catastrophic injuries at the Hillsborough football stadium when the grandstand collapsed and was subsequently in a PVS for over three years.

On 4 February 1993, the highest court in the country ruled that the feeding tube that was keeping Anthony Bland alive should be removed and he should be allowed to die. Thus, the Lords confirmed that in certain circumstances it is acceptable to withdraw life-sustaining treatments. However, in each case of withdrawal of artificial nutrition and hydration, an application to the courts has to be made until sufficient experience has been amassed to negate the individual application.

Patients in PVS can survive for years, or even decades, in this non-autonomous state. It is very distressing for the patient's relatives and is considered by some to be undignified for the patient. There are generally two schools of thought regarding the withdrawal of treatment from such patients. Pro-lifers would argue that if patients are insentient, they will not be aware that they are living a life of no quality and therefore there is no reason to end it. Hence, by withdrawing artificial nutrition and hydration (effectively starvation, of which the patient will not be aware), death occurs and would be a great harm, which is in direct opposition to the principle of non-maleficence.

Those who believe withdrawal of treatment (passive euthanasia) to let the patient die, the kindest course of action, would do so in the belief that they are acting beneficently because maintaining a life of such poor quality is in fact the greater harm and death would therefore, not be harmful and indeed, be a benefit. Artificial nutrition and hydration in the case of the patient with PVS does not appear to be futile as it is doing exactly what it is meant to do, i.e. keeping the patient alive. It cannot, therefore, be withdrawn on grounds of futility unless it is considered that maintaining the life is futile.

EUTHANASIA

Euthanasia literally means 'good death' and is often referred to as 'mercy killing'. However, euthanasia is in fact the intentional killing of a human being, either through act or omission, for the benefit of the patient. The definition of murder is 'intentionally killing', therefore in the UK, euthanasia is equivalent to murder and thus illegal. Euthanasia may take several forms: passive or active, voluntary, involuntary or non-voluntary.

Passive euthanasia, also known as euthanasia by omission, is generally considered to be 'letting die', which involves the withdrawal of active treatment or withholding life-sustaining treatments which may be of benefit to the patient and therefore the patient dies through this intentional omission. This should not be confused with the withholding or withdrawal of treatments that are considered to be ineffective and therefore futile, even though they may prolong the process of dying. The patient will therefore die from the medical condition from which he or she is suffering. This course of action frequently takes place in healthcare settings and is legally endorsed when carried out appropriately.

Active euthanasia refers to the taking of direct action to end a patient's life, for example administering a lethal injection, and is illegal. However, it is not illegal to administer high doses of drugs to ensure a terminally ill patient is kept pain-free, even if it is clear that the drugs will shorten life, as long as the intention is to kill the pain, not the patient (see Doctrine of double effect).

If euthanasia is voluntary, the patient has requested it. If it is involuntary, it is against the patient's wishes, and if it is non-voluntary, it is without the patient's consent because he or she lacks capacity.

The laws regarding euthanasia are reviewed periodically and are subject to much debate. The main argument for euthanasia to be decriminalised is the patient's 'right to die'. However, if the law were to be changed, it is also the doctor's 'right to kill' that would be granted because it would mean one person could facilitate the death of another. Those against euthanasia argue that those who work in what is essentially a caring profession should not wish to kill, nor indeed be legally sanctioned to do so.

Arguments for euthanasia

- It provides a course of action to alleviate extreme pain and suffering and would therefore be viewed as a beneficent act. Supporters of euthanasia argue that there is a moral duty to respect the wishes of the patient with terminal illness or incurable suffering who wishes to die.
- It provides a course of action to end a life not worth living because quality of life is so low; it is a burden and again would be viewed as a beneficent act.
- Resources can be diverted to people who may achieve more benefit, which would provide a more just allocation of resources.
- It allows freedom of choice, thereby enhancing autonomy in end-of-life decisions. The principles of autonomy, liberty of choice and self-determination are central to the classic 'right to die' arguments.

Arguments against euthanasia

- It devalues the sanctity of human life and is therefore a maleficent action.
- The 'slippery slope' effect, i.e. if A is allowed to happen, it will soon follow that B or even C will happen. Accepting the act in question would cross a line that has already been drawn against killing; and once that line has been crossed, it will not be possible to draw it again to preclude unacceptable acts and practices (Beauchamp & Childress, 2001).
- Doctors should not be involved in directly causing the death of patients in their care.
- Euthanasia could be viewed as a means to cost containment within health care.

CONCLUSION

In this chapter, an overview to the ethical issues associated with dying and death has been discussed. The major ethical theories and principles have been outlined and the concept of medical futility has been discussed. The principles of acting in the best interests of the patient have been outlined, together with the ethics of withholding and withdrawing active treatment. The ethical concerns surrounding PVS and the ethical concepts of euthanasia have been discussed.

REFERENCES

Airedale NHS Trust v Bland [1993] AC 789.

Beauchamp TL, Childress JF (2001) *Principles of Biomedical Ethics*, 5th edn. Oxford University Press, Oxford.

British Medical Association, Resuscitation Council (UK) and Royal College of Nursing (2007) *Decisions relating to cardiopulmonary resuscitation: A joint statement from the British Medical Association, the Resuscitation Council (UK) and the Royal College of Nursing*. Available at www.resus. org.uk/pages/dnar.pdf (accessed July 2009).

Bowker L, Stewart K (1999) Predicting unsuccessful cardiopulmonary resuscitation (CPR): A comparison of three morbidity scores. *Resuscitation* **40**: 89–95.

Braddock CH (1999) Termination of life-sustaining treatment. Available at www.dets.washington.edu/bioethx/topics/termlife.html (accessed 25 November 2007).

British Medical Association (BMA) (1996) *Treatment Decisions for Patients in Persistent Vegetative State*. Available at www.bma.org.uk/ap.nsf/Content/pvs (accessed 12 December 2007).

Department for Constitutional Affairs (2005) *Mental Capacity Act*. TSO, London.

De Wolf Bosek MS, Savage TA (2007) *The Ethical Component of Nursing Education: Integrating Ethics into Clinical Experience*. Lippincott, London.

Devettere RJ (2000) *Practical Decision Making in Health Care Ethics: Cases and Concepts*. Georgetown University Press, Washington.

Department of Health (DH) (2001) *Reference Guide to Consent for Examination or Treatment*. HMSO, London.

Ewanchuck M, Brindley PG (2006) Ethics review: Perioperative do-not-resuscitate orders – doing 'nothing' when something can be done. Available at www.ccforum.com (accessed 15 April 2007).

Fletcher L, Buka P (1999) *A Legal Framework for Caring: An Introduction to Law and Ethics in Heath Care*. Macmillan, London.

Glover J (1977) The sanctity of life. In: *Bioethics: An Anthology* (eds H Khuse & P Singer), 2nd edn. Blackwell Publishing, Oxford.

Jecker NS (2000) Futility. Available at www.depts.washington.edu/bioethx/topics/futil.html (accessed 27 April 2007).y

Nursing and Midwifery Council (NMC) (2002) *Code of Professional Conduct*. NMC, London.

Rachels J (1975) Active and opassive euthanasia. In: *Bioethics: An Anthology* (eds H Khuse & P Singer) (2006), 2nd edn, Blackwell Publishing, Oxford.

Wacker Guido G (2006). *Legal and Ethical Issues in Nursing*, 4th edn. Pearson Prentice Hall, New Jersey.

5 Complementary Therapies in Palliative Care

Rachel McGuinness

INTRODUCTION

Complementary therapies can be provided alongside, and in conjunction with, orthodox medical treatment; alternative therapies are therapies provided in place of orthodox medical treatment (British Medical Association (BMA), 1993) (cited in Kohn & Maher, 2006).

In this chapter, the use of complementary therapies that are most commonly used within palliative care settings will be discussed, with particular focus on those that may be more appropriate to the needs of the dying patient, e.g. aromatherapy, massage and reflexology. These therapies are based on the humanistic model, requiring either physical application or having psychological effects.

The aim of this chapter is to understand the principles of complementary therapies in palliative care.

LEARNING OUTCOMES

At the end of this chapter, the reader will be able to:

❑ Discuss the classification of complementary and alternative therapies.
❑ List the goals of complementary therapies.
❑ Discuss the holistic approach of complementary therapies.
❑ Outline the role of complementary therapy in symptom control.
❑ Describe the principles of the use of complementary therapies commonly used in palliative care.
❑ Outline the referral process for complementary therapies.

CLASSIFICATION OF COMPLEMENTARY AND ALTERNATIVE THERAPIES

In order to understand the role of complementary and alternative therapies in the end-of-life setting, it is important to understand the classification of the different therapies under the umbrella term 'complementary and alternative medicine'.

Therapies have been classified and grouped in a variety of ways. For example, the House of Lords Report (2000) groups complementary and alternative therapies into two categories according to their professional regulation and evidence base (Table 5.1).

Table 5.1 Categorising of complementary and alternative therapies (Adapted from House of Lords Report, 2000)

Professionally organised alternative therapies	Complementary therapies
• Acupuncture • Chiropractic • Herbal medicine • Homoeopathy • Osteopathy	• Alexander technique • Aromatherapy • Bach and other flower remedies • Bodywork therapies including massage • Counselling stress therapy • Hypnotherapy • Reflexology • Meditation • Shiatsu • Healing • Marharishi ayurvedic medicine • Nutritional medicine • Yoga

These groups may then be classified on the basis of their application, for example:

• Physical application, e.g. massage or other touch therapies.
• Psychological effect, e.g. relaxation techniques, guided imagery and visualisation.
• Pharmacological basis, e.g. dietary supplements.

(Kohn & Maher, 2006)

Other classifications of complementary therapies look at the humanistic and radical holistic model in which the humanistic model aims to provide support, relief and/or reduction in symptoms/side-effects of treatments and to maintain quality of life for patients. It is this model that forms the basis of those therapies used within the NHS and palliative care. The radical holistic model encompasses the theory of self-healing approaches for those hoping to achieve increased survival and possible cure; this model is not advocated within the NHS (Kohn, 1999).

Howells (1997, cited in Kohn, 1999) suggests therapies may also be classified by how they are provided to the patient, for example they may be provided by hospital-based practitioners within a multidisciplinary approach or through external approaches used by the NHS.

However, there is also a great deal of evidence on the use of acupuncture with palliative care, which may also be of benefit to patients at the end of life. Other therapies suggested under 'Professionally organised alternative therapies' and 'Complementary therapies' of the House of Lords report may also be used within this field.

GOALS OF COMPLEMENTARY THERAPIES

Most complementary therapies follow a philosophy that is consistent with the goals of palliative care and the needs of palliative care patients (Deegan, 2006). One of the reasons for this may be due to the direct similarities in their goals; Table 5.2 demonstrates these similarities and why they could work together side by side.

Table 5.2 Similarities between the goals of palliative care and complementary therapies

Goals/service	Palliative care	Complementary therapies
Improve quality of life	Yes	Yes
Provide relief from pain and other symptoms	Yes	Yes
Integrate psychological and spiritual aspects of care	Yes	Yes
Offer support to patient and family	Yes	Yes

HOLISTIC APPROACH OF COMPLEMENTARY THERAPIES

'Dying people require a truly holistic approach to their care' (Faull & Nyatanga, 2005).

The underlying philosophy of complementary therapies is to treat every individual as a whole, encompassing all aspects of their physical, emotional, social and spiritual needs. The concept that every individual is unique and needs to be treated accordingly is also extremely important. One of the reasons for the increased use of complementary therapies in palliative care may be the continuing attention to the psychological, emotional and spiritual needs of dying people (Reoch, 1997).

The additional use of complementary therapies may help to ensure that patients feel cared for, they may benefit from the time that the therapist can offer them to listen and support them, and to develop the therapeutic relationship between the patient and therapist. This may help them at times when patients may feel isolated or alone.

There is also the consideration that within the philosophy of complementary therapies there is a continuing positive approach, and it is never the case that there is 'nothing more that can be done for the patient' (Deegan, 2006). This approach lends itself well to the considerations of caring for the dying patient as it suggests that despite there being no cure, there are still ways in which the patient may be able to help themselves to feel better.

COMPLEMENTARY THERAPY IN SYMPTOM CONTROL

Complementary therapies are used frequently within palliative care to complement and improve symptom control (Deegan, 2006). An article in *Michigan Nurse* (Teaching notes, 2000) suggests that the most prevalent symptoms experienced by dying individuals are pain, dyspnoea, nausea, vomiting, fear, anxiety and delirium, and that when the patient is recognised to be dying, the most relevant clinical goal is to palliate symptoms of distress.

Complementary therapies may be helpful in relieving some of these symptoms, particularly attempting to relieve symptoms of distress through inducing relaxation, but evidence also suggests that certain complementary therapies may be useful in reducing pain, and in helping to reduce fear and anxiety. However, it is apparent that further research into the benefits of complementary therapies is required.

It is also important to understand here the concept of touch during this time and how this can play an important part in care. Patients at palliative or end stage in their disease process may feel that their body is no longer capable of experiencing pleasant feelings, and the application of gentle massage or touch may help them to realise this is still possible. This emphasis on physical touch can sometimes be absent in a more intensive conventional medical setting (Deegan, 2006). There is sometimes a sense of fear or awkwardness of contact between carers and the patient, and the inclusion of touch may help to relieve this. In this case it may be possible for the carer to be shown some gentle massage to encourage this interaction. An example of this is demonstrated in Scenarios 5.1 and 5.2.

PRINCIPLES OF THE USE OF COMPLEMENTARY THERAPIES COMMONLY USED IN PALLIATIVE CARE

The following are examples of complementary therapies that are being used within the field of palliative care with cancer patients and may be particularly beneficial in end-of-life care; the case studies demonstrate how they may be used. Each of these therapies involves an initial assessment with the patient in order to identify individual needs and any contra-indications and, as with all complementary therapies, requires informed consent from the patient.

Aromatherapy

Aromatherapy is a holistic therapy that involves the use of essential oils. These essential oils are extracted from various parts of plants, including roots, leaves, flowers or fruits, and can be used in a variety of ways according to the needs of the patient.

The initial consultation with the patient determines what method of treatment is the most appropriate, and suitable essential oils will be chosen to help with the specific symptoms. In the case of palliative care and end of life, the following methods may be used where appropriate.

Massage
Massage therapy alone is a system of treatment of the soft tissue of the body, involving kneading, stroking and in some cases an element of pressure to various parts of the body with the aim of alleviating the aches, pains and musculoskeletal problems sometimes associated with tension.

The massage used in aromatherapy is very gentle and involves a blend of essential oils combined with carrier oil. Massage may be given to the back, neck and shoulders, hands and arms or feet and legs. Oils may be chosen to help with relaxation, to provide pain relief or assist with reducing anxiety.

Compression
A blend of oils may be applied directly to specific areas of pain or inflammation.

Inhalation
A single essential oil or blend of oils may be given to inhale from a tissue. This may be given in cases of anxiety or breathlessness (Cooper, 2007).

Vaporisation
Essential oils may be diffused in a room to help the patient, for example in the case of unpleasant odours as a result of fungating wounds. This may help in promoting a more pleasant environment for patients and their family or carers (Johns, 2004; Cooper, 2007).

Creams and lotions
A specific blend of essential oils may be combined within a lotion base for symptoms that may not be responding to medical treatment, for example itching skin complaints or to help with pain relief.

Scenario 5.1 Aromatherapy/ massage

Matthew, a 37-year-old man with non-Hodgkin's lymphoma, was referred for complementary therapy by his psychologist as he was very tearful and 'prone to shaking' due to anxiety. His initial referral was to be seen at an outpatient clinic, but Mathew's condition deteriorated rapidly and he was admitted to hospital.

As a result of his cancer treatment there were serious complications, which resulted in damage to his heart, and after each course of treatment his condition was very weak and he was extremely breathless. The complexities of his condition and continuing treatment meant that he remained in hospital for the next couple of months, only going home for one or two days at the most.

Matthew was very keen to receive some massage to his back to help him relax, so ward visits were carried out once or twice a week in order to provide massage at the bedside. Aromatherapy oils were chosen to help him with relaxation and anxiety, but were also considered for helping with breathlessness. A topical lotion blend was also provided for relief of itching skin.

Matthew had described feeling very low in mood most days but commented that he always looked forward to his massages and the relief it gave him; he often felt so relaxed afterwards that he would sleep for a couple of hours following the session. Matthew also felt the aromatherapy sessions helped him to cope better with the side-effects of his treatment, as well as helping him to cope with his anxieties and fears. Over the sessions with the therapist, Matthew often shared his thoughts and fears on how he felt about dying and gradually began to show signs of acceptance about this.

Matthew's wife was pleased to see how much he was benefiting from the sessions and asked if she could be shown how to provide massage for him. Sessions were arranged to show her some simple massage skills, and a blend of oils was given for her to use. Both Matthew and his wife found this to be very rewarding and she enjoyed being able to help him in this way during her visits.

Matthew continued to receive aromatherapy massage over the last few weeks of his life from both the therapist and his wife, who had also begun to receive therapies at an outpatient clinic for her support as a carer.

Reflexology

Reflexology involves the therapist applying precise use of 'touch' or appropriate pressure to various points on the feet or in some cases the hands. These specific areas or 'reflex' points are thought to correspond to the rest of the body, and therefore working on these areas aims to promote relaxation and maintain homeostasis within the rest of the body.

Reflexology is not just a massage but a powerful system of health care, useful for achieving and maintaining health and enhancing well-being, as well as for relieving symptoms or causes of illness and disease (Mackareth, 2002).

Reflexology is a non-invasive therapy that can be adapted to meet the needs of the individual with limited resources, making it appropriate to a variety of settings.

Scenario 5.2 Reflexology

Sharon, a 52-year-old lady with breast cancer and liver and lung metastases, was referred for complementary therapy by her GP. Sharon was undergoing chemotherapy treatment and was feeling extremely anxious, very low in mood and experiencing pain, breathlessness and fatigue. After an initial consultation, Sharon decided to try reflexology and began to attend one of our outpatient clinics.

It became clear after her first couple of sessions that Sharon's condition was deteriorating, and attending her appointments was becoming difficult. It was arranged for Sharon to receive a home visit on a weekly basis in order for her to continue with reflexology as she felt it was helping her to cope better by giving her a sense of peace, helping her to relax and let go of her feelings of anxiety.

Sharon's family were also very supportive and were keen to become involved and wanted to do whatever they could to help her to relax and feel comforted.

They had already started to give her gentle massage at home, which she enjoyed. So we provided them with an essential oil blend for their use with gentle and relaxing aromatherapy oils and showed them further massage skills. They continued

Continued

---

to provide gentle massage, accompanied by soothing music, to her feet and head on a regular basis. Sharon benefited from this caring experience immensely and the family felt some comfort in knowing they were able to help her in this way.

The therapist continued to visit on a weekly basis for the next four weeks, providing gentle reflexology and foot massages at the bedside and offering support for the patient and family up until the final week of Sharon's life.

Reiki

Reiki is a very gentle, non-invasive therapy that involves the therapist placing his or her hands on or directly above various points along the body. Reiki is a Japanese term that translates as 'universal life force energy'; its gentle approach aims to achieve a sense of well-being and balance within the mind and body.

Evidence suggests that Reiki and spiritual healing may help to promote relaxation, provide emotional/spiritual support, promote well-being, reduce tension and stress, contribute to pain relief, improve sleep, reduce the side-effects of chemotherapy and radiotherapy, and support the patient in the dying process (Kohn & Maher, 2006) (Scenario 5.3).

Scenario 5.3 Reiki

Ernie, an 82-year-old man, was diagnosed with cancer of the colon and lung, with multiple bone metastases, and was at end stage. He was referred for complementary therapy by his Macmillan nurse during his stay in hospital and was in need of support for anxiety and depression. Ernie was very weak and experiencing pain in his groin and legs, and had recently received palliative radiotherapy for pain control to the bone metastases in his shoulder, knee, foot and arm. Ernie described feeling very low in mood and also expressed that he felt very isolated and alone due to being on a side ward with little opportunity for social interaction. Ernie had been in hospital for the past six weeks and was very keen to return to his nursing home.

Due to the complexities of Ernie's multiple bone metastases, certain therapies were not appropriate; however, it was clear that Ernie needed some help and support at this time and was keen to try anything that would help him to feel better. It was suggested to Ernie that Reiki would be a suitable option due to the extremely gentle nature of the therapy and after an explanation of what was involved Ernie agreed.

A 20-min Reiki session was given while Ernie lay comfortably in his hospital bed, with the added use of relaxing music. Following the session, Ernie described feeling very relaxed and described the session as 'very warm' and 'soothing'. When asked, Ernie was keen to receive a return visit the following week.

At this point Ernie was transferred back to his nursing home and was subsequently offered to continue his sessions there, to which he agreed.

A further three visits were carried out at the nursing home once a week for the last few weeks of Ernie's life at his request. At each visit Ernie received Reiki for 15–20 min and continued to benefit from the relaxation and feeling of calmness that each session gave him, often falling asleep at the end of each session.

Relaxation and visualisation/guided imagery

The act of 'stilling the mind' can lead to a reduction in worry and psychological stress, and this connection between mind and body is an area that is becoming increasingly recognised through the field of psychoneuroimmunology (Kohn, 1999).

Visualisation and guided imagery focus on the use of mental pictures (such as a peaceful scene) in order to calm and relax the mind. Together with relaxation techniques for controlled breathing and relaxing the body, patients may benefit from a reduction in symptoms such as pain, nausea and vomiting (Deegan, 2006). Such techniques may be used with the patient at the end of life to relieve such symptoms as well as anxiety and distress.

REFERRAL PROCESS FOR COMPLEMENTARY THERAPIES

Patients and carers should be able to self-refer, or have a family member or health professional refer them for assessment for

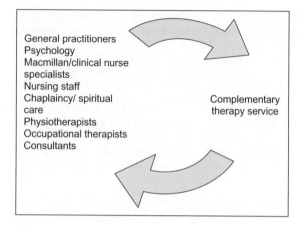

General practitioners
Psychology
Macmillan/clinical nurse
specialists
Nursing staff
Chaplaincy/ spiritual
care
Physiotherapists
Occupational therapists
Consultants

Complementary
therapy service

Fig 5.1 Examples of who can refer to the complementary therapy service.

complementary therapies (Kohn & Maher, 2006). Although access and the referral process vary according to the individual service provider, irrespective of who refers to a complementary therapy service, access to information on complementary therapies should be made available to all those involved in the care of the patient in order to ensure that the needs of the patient will be recognised. The complementary therapy service can receive referrals from a variety of sources (Fig. 5.1).

Referral criteria are necessary in order to recognise where complementary therapies may be appropriate and form a good basis for the understanding between complementary therapists and other healthcare professionals.

It is important to recognise the need for an integrated and multidisciplinary approach in order to identify and fulfil the needs of the patient. Communication between healthcare professionals and complementary therapists is extremely important to provide quality care. Complementary therapists are required to document, evaluate and communicate with the multidisciplinary team and also to refer to other healthcare professionals when required (Mackareth & Carter, 2006). The complementary therapies service at Walsall Primary Care Trust (Box 5.1) is fully integrated into the field of palliative care, demonstrating a multidisciplinary approach to complementary therapy provision.

Box 5.1 Complementary therapy services at Walsall Primary Care Trust

This service began in 1993 and offers complementary therapies free of charge to patients requiring palliative and supportive cancer care across the borough of Walsall. Its structure enables patients to access complementary therapies in various settings: outpatient clinics, domiciliary visits and an inpatient service for Walsall's Manor Hospital.

The involvement of the service requires referral from healthcare professionals and provides guidelines and referral criteria for its use. Its aim is to offer support and aid symptom control for patients at all stages of their diagnosis and disease progression and at end of life, at the location that is most suitable to their needs. The service offers aromatherapy, massage, reflexology, reiki and relaxation for patients and carers.

The service also consists of a complementary therapy committee, which regularly reports to the palliative care strategy group. Its structure ensures a multidisciplinary approach and delivers education on complementary therapies to other healthcare professionals at regular intervals.

CONCLUSION

This chapter has provided an overview to the principles of complementary therapies in palliative care. The classification of complementary and alternative therapies has been outlined. Goals of complementary therapies have been listed and the holistic approach to complementary therapies has been discussed. The role of complementary therapy in symptom control has been described and the principles of the use of complementary therapies commonly used in palliative care discussed.

REFERENCES

Cooper E (2007) Palliative and supportive care. In: *Aromatherapy for Health Professionals* (eds S Price & L Price), 3rd edn. Churchill Livingstone, USA.

Deegan T (2006) Complementary therapies in palliative care. In: *Primary Palliative Care, Dying, Death and Bereavement in the Community* (ed. R Charlton). Radcliffe Medical Press, Oxford.

Faull C, Nyatanga B (2005) Terminal care and dying. In: *Handbook of Palliative Care* (eds C Faull, Y Carter, L Daniels), 2nd edn. Blackwell Publishing, India.

House of Lords (2000) *Science and Technology, Sixth Report.* London: Publications Parliament. Available at. www.publications.parliament.uk (accessed 30 November 2007).

Johns C (2004) *Being Mindful, Easing Suffering, Reflections on Palliative Care.* Jessica Kingsley Publishers, London.

Kohn M (1999) *Complementary Therapies in Cancer Care: An Abridged Report of a Study Produced for Macmillan Cancer Relief.* Macmillan Cancer Relief, London.

Kohn M, Maher J (2006) *ABC of Palliative Care*, 2nd edn. BMJ Books, Singapore.

Mackareth PA, Carter A (2006) *Massage and Bodywork: Adapting Therapies for Cancer Care.* Churchill Livingstone, London.

Mackareth PA (2002) *Clinical Reflexology, A Guide for Health Professionals.* Churchill Livingstone, London.

Reoch R (1997) *Dying Well, A Holistic Guide for the Dying and their Carers.* Gaia Books Limited, London.

Teaching notes (2000) Symptom management strategies for dying patients. *Michigan Nurse* **73**(1): 10–17.

SUGGESTED FURTHER READING

Autton N (1996) The use of touch in palliative care. *Eur J Palliative Care* **3**: 121–124.

Correa-Velez I, Clavarino A, Barnett A, Eastwood H (2003) Use of complementary and alternative medicine and quality of life: changes at the end of life. *J Palliative Med* **17**: 695–703.

Filshie J (2000) Acupuncture in palliative care. *Eur J Palliative Care* **7**: 41–44.

Gordon J, Curtins S (2000) *Comprehensive Cancer Care: Integrating Alternative and Conventional Therapies.* Perseus Publishing, London.

Kubler R (1969) *On Death and Dying.* Touchstone, New York.

McCabe P (2001) *Complementary Therapies in Nursing and Midwifery: From Vision to Practice.* Ausmed Publications, Melbourne.

Mitchell A, Cormack M (1999) *The Therapeutic Relationship in Complementary Health Care.* Churchill Livingstone, London.

Ronaldson S (2000) *Spirituality, The Heart of Nursing.* Ausmed Publications, Melbourne.

Tavares M (2003a) *The National Guidelines for the Use of Complementary Therapies in Supportive & Palliative Care*. The Prince of Wales's Foundation for Integrated Health, London.

Tavares M (2003b) *New Guidelines for the Use of Complementary Therapies for People with Life Threatening Illnesses*. Press Release, London.

Useful websites and addresses

For further information on complementary therapies and integrated healthcare, visit the website: www.fih.org.uk or contact The Prince's Foundation for Integrated Health, 33–41 Dallington Street, London, EC1V 0BB. Tel 020 3119 3100.

National Association of Complementary Therapists in Hospice and Palliative Care, 32 Milner Road, Selly Park, Birmingham, B29 7RQ. Tel: 0121 472 4987.

6 | Relatives Witnessing Resuscitation

Melanie Humphreys

INTRODUCTION

There are an estimated 25 000 to 30 000 resuscitation attempts in the UK every year (Royal College of Nursing (RCN), 2004). The specialist areas that are most likely to be involved are emergency departments and critical care areas. Dealing with the relatives of a patient during a resuscitation situation can be difficult for all staff involved, regardless of their experience.

Relatives witnessing resuscitation is the process of active medical resuscitation in the presence of family members; it is becoming more common in the in-hospital setting after published studies demonstrated clear benefits for relatives. However, approval of relatives witnessing resuscitation is not universal amongst all healthcare professionals. Concerns have been raised regarding the potential for family members' presence to affect the performance of the team and possibly interfere with the patient (Weslien *et al.*, 2006); witnessing the attempt can be traumatic and have a negative emotional and psychological consequence (Crisci, 1994; Fein *et al.*, 2004). In addition, the witnessing of resuscitation has some ethical and medicolegal implications (Boyd, 2000).

The aim of this chapter is to understand the issues surrounding relatives witnessing resuscitation.

LEARNING OUTCOMES

At the end of this chapter, the reader will be able to:

❏ Discuss the historical background to relatives witnessing resuscitation.
❏ Discuss the perceived advantages and disadvantages of relatives witnessing resuscitation.

HISTORICAL BACKGROUND TO RELATIVES WITNESSING RESUSCITATION

The notion of relatives witnessing resuscitation was first reported during the 1980s through work within the Foote Hospital, Michigan (Doyle *et al.*, 1987). The practice came about as the result of a request from two family members to remain with their relative during resuscitation efforts; this resulted in the introduction of a structured programme that enabled family members to be with their relative during cardiopulmonary resuscitation (CPR). A subsequent evaluation of 47 respondents who had been present revealed:

- 36 (77%) believed that their adjustment to the death was made easier by witnessing CPR of their relative.
- 30 (64%) believed that their presence had been beneficial to the patient.
- 44 (94%) would choose to attend if the situation ever arose again.

A survey with 21 members of the emergency staff indicated that although 6 (29%) reported some added stress, 71% endorsed continuation of the practice. Nine years after the inception of the programme, Hanson & Strawser (1992) reported that distressed family members made no attempt to interfere during CPR, the biggest reported concern of healthcare professionals opposing the process; this has been further supported in more recent studies (Boyd, 2000). Other concerns centre around possible complaints regarding apparent weaknesses in the medical treatment and that the presence of family members could increase the stress on healthcare professionals (Weslien *et al.*, 2006).

DETERMINING BEST INTEREST

The decision to enable family members to be present during a resuscitation attempt should be made in the best interests of the person who is being resuscitated. When the person who is being resuscitated is not able to communicate his or her wishes or has not previously expressed their wishes in an advance directive (discussed further in Chapter 4), the decision about who should be present during resuscitation should be made jointly by members of the resuscitation team and family members. In this regard, discussion should be facilitated by experienced health-care professionals. When appropriate, spiritual leaders or other trained members of the healthcare team may assume this role (Fulbrook *et al.*, 2007). Whilst this position seems plausible, it is very difficult in reality, as a healthcare professional, to be certain of which choice is indeed in each individual patient's best interest. Of course, if the patient who is being resuscitated has expressed a prior wish, this should always be respected. Because of the multiculturally diverse environment in which practition-ers work, the resuscitation team should also take the individual patient's and family's beliefs, values and rituals into account. The patient's and the family's cultural background should be assessed with respect to the provision of appropriate individual-ised care.

The motive is that a holistic care approach might support family members through the critical event (Goldsworth, 1998). According to this, the family members are allowed to come close, have the opportunity to see, talk and touch their relative, and are supervised at all times (Eichhorn *et al.*, 2001). The importance is emphasised to show respect for the decisions made by the family without blaming any of its members for deciding whether or not to be present (Weslien *et al.*, 2006).

In a replica study to the Foote Hospital one (Doyle *et al.*, 1987), Meyers *et al.* (1998) reported that 80% of relatives would have wanted to be present during CPR had they been given the option, believing that their presence might have helped their family member (this compares favourably with the Foote Hospital study). It does appear that there is increasing pressure on practi-tioners to facilitate this process. Indeed, all major organisations concerned with resuscitation have issued guidelines recom-mending that, where appropriate, the witnessing of resuscitation should be enabled (Resuscitation Council UK, 1996; American Heart Association in collaboration with the International Liaison Committee on Resuscitation (AHA & ILCOR), 2000; Baskett *et al.*, 2005; Fulbrook *et al.*, 2007).

However, not all studies report witnessing as the favoured option; it is worth considering that Grice *et al.* (2003) found that the majority of the patients who were to undergo heart or vas-cular surgery did not want their family members to be present during a possible resuscitation. The authors also found that about half of the same family members did not want to be present. There have been many factors since the 1980s that have shaped attitudes favouring relatives witnessing resuscitation, but of fundamental importance are the views of survivors of the arrest and their relatives. It is only on the gathering of data from a significant body of survivors that the determination of the decision made by healthcare professionals – on their behalf – that a judgement can be made. To date, the number of studies that has investigated the viewpoints of cardiac arrest survivors whose family has been present is minimal. One such study was undertaken on four patients who had undergone CPR and survived; each reported they were comfortable with the presence of family members (Eichhorn *et al.*, 2001). Clearly, this is a very limited sample and further research with these groups is necessary to complete the missing gaps in knowledge and understanding.

The most recent position guidelines published, which are a joint statement from the European Federation of Critical Care Nursing associations (EfCCNa), the European Society of Paediatric and Neonatal Intensive Care (ESPNIC) and the European Society of Cardiology Council on Cardiovascular Nursing and Allied Professions Joint Position Statement (CCNAP) (Fulbrook *et al.*, 2007), state that:

- All patients have the right to have family members present during resuscitation.
- The patient's family members should be offered the opportunity to be present during resuscitation of a relative.
- Support should be provided by an appropriately qualified healthcare professional whose responsibility is to care for family members witnessing CPR.
- Professional counselling should be offered to family members who have witnessed a resuscitation event.
- All members of the resuscitation team who were involved in a resuscitation attempt when family members were present should participate in team debriefing.
- Family presence during resuscitation should be incorporated into the curricula of CPR training programmes.

- All intensive and critical care units should have multidisciplinary written guidelines on the presence of family members during CPR.

These guidelines concur with previous significant position statements (Resuscitation Council UK, 1996; Baskett *et al.*, 2005). In the light of guidelines presented, it is always appropriate that practitioners evaluate individual family members, e.g. their coping strategies, mental stability and behaviour. Some family members could, for instance, be inclined to violence or be under the influence of drugs. Therefore, when considering patients' best interests, it is necessary that practitioners are available to assess the appropriateness of each of the family members to be present in order for them to have a fulfilling role within the resuscitation room (Weslien *et al.*, 2006). Indeed, it is an opportunity to be assured that everything has been done for their loved one, which may have a positive effect in an eventual grieving process, as reported in many studies (Meyers *et al.*, 1998), regardless of the predicted outcome (Mazer *et al.*, 2006).

IMPORTANCE OF PATIENT CONFIDENTIALITY

A patient's permission is required before medical information may be disclosed to a third party. This assurance of confidentiality creates a bond of trust that encourages patients to disclose personal information to healthcare professionals. It has been argued that allowing relatives into the resuscitation room can be seen as ignoring the patient's right to confidentiality, and those who breach this confidentiality could find themselves the subject of disciplinary action or possible litigation (Stewart & Bowker, 1997). Stewart & Bowker further state that between a quarter and a third of patients do not seem to want their relatives involved in decisions regarding whether resuscitation should be attempted, and believe that it is unlikely that these patients would want their relatives to witness the actual procedure. In response to this claim, McLauchlan (1997), Chairman of the Resuscitation Council Project Team, argued that the risks, although correct, are outweighed by the potential benefit to the relative or close friend.

To date, this remains a theoretical discussion as no complaint has yet been brought before any of the statutory bodies, such as the Nursing and Midwifery Council (NMC) or the General Medical Council (GMC).

Patients will often ask doctors to share clinical details with a relative or friend, but for adults there is no automatic right to this, and practitioners should obtain the patient's permission before discussing their clinical condition with others. Patients who are unconscious or gravely ill have the same rights to confidentiality as conscious patients, but it is, of course, impossible to obtain their views. In these circumstances, Stewart & Bowker (1997) argue strongly that doctors cannot assume that patients would consent to their relatives witnessing their treatment. It needs to be borne in mind, however, that when a patient is unable to communicate, relatives may be invaluable in providing additional medical information.

From a legal viewpoint, relatives in the UK have no legal rights in the care of adult patients. However, a recent trend towards increased patient autonomy has altered the views of patients and relatives towards acute care provision (RCN, 2004). Many relatives will have been present at pre-hospital resuscitation attempts and witnessed resuscitation. Fundamentally, obtaining a patient's consent to allow relatives into the resuscitation room will often be impossible, although any known pre-existing wishes of the patient must be respected. It is a general and ethical principle that valid consent must be obtained on every occasion when a healthcare professional wishes to initiate treatment or any other intervention, except in emergencies or where the law states otherwise. This principle reflects the rights of patients to determine what happens to their own bodies and is a fundamental part of good practice (Department of Health (DH), 2001). Courts are increasingly recognising the power of advance directives or 'living wills' (discussed further in Chapter 10).

EFFECT ON THE GRIEVING PROCESS
In terms of the effects on the relative witnessing the process, whilst many studies report a therapeutic effect (Grice *et al.*, 2003; Fulbrook *et al.*, 2005; Gold *et al.*, 2006), healthcare professionals need to be ever-mindful of the deleterious effects – these can be considered to be some of the most powerful and persuasive to the doubters of this process (van der Woning, 1999; Walker,

2006). Arguments are posed surrounding the unknown long-term effects of witnessing such traumatic events on a loved one. Indeed, some of the more recent UK-based studies, although small and biased toward emergency departments, are still showing reticence towards introducing the process. Back & Rooke (1994) reported in their survey that 13 (65% of study participants) had experience of a family member being present during CPR, but only seven reported a positive encounter. Reasons for a negative encounter remain largely unexplored. In this survey, they reported that 15 (75%) would allow family members to be present during resuscitation only if escorted by an experienced member of staff – this is, without doubt, a very commonsense approach. All the guidelines offered are very clear regarding the presence of an experienced healthcare professional remaining with the relatives at all times, guiding them through the process and removing them from the room should the need arise (Resuscitation Council UK, 1996; AHA & ILCOR, 2000; Fulbrook, *et al.*, 2007). Indeed, in some of the studies that have reported negative outcomes for the witnessing relative, such outcomes have been due to this omission (Osuagwu, 1991; Goldstein, *et al.*, 1997; van der Woning, 1999), clearly suggesting that if such a person is not available to offer this support then the chances of this initiative being helpful and fulfilling are vastly reduced.

However, Fulbrook *et al.* (2007) concede that on occasions when it may not be possible to provide a healthcare professional whose sole responsibility is to care for the family member, this should not mean the exclusion of the family member from the resuscitation. Rather, an experienced member of the resuscitation team, who is not undertaking a lead role, should be designated as primarily responsible for the continued care of the family member.

Practitioners are clearly very concerned about the possibility of long-term negative psychological effects resulting from witnessing resuscitation (Fulbrook, *et al.*, 2005). In the study undertaken by Robinson *et al.* (1998), it was concluded that relatives who remained in the resuscitation room were no more distressed by their experience than those who were kept in a nearby relatives' room. Furthermore, when assessed three months after the event, there was a trend towards lower degrees of intrusive imagery, post-traumatic avoidance behaviour and symptoms of grief in the relatives who had witnessed the procedure. Within this small study group, both groups were bereaved, but it is true to say that the additional psychiatric effect of witnessing resuscitation is difficult to predict in such small-scale studies. Interestingly, based on current available knowledge, no guidelines or similar recommendations have been found that advocate that family members should *not* be present during resuscitation.

It is worth considering who should initiate discussion around the possibility of witnessing resuscitation. In a USA-based study undertaken by Meyers *et al.* (1998), an overwhelming 96% of families believed that individuals have the right to be present if they so desire. These findings underscore the basic beliefs of the sample regarding the wholeness and integrity of the family unit at the time of death, which are that, whenever possible, needs should be respected and supported rather than opposed. In the study by Back & Rooke (1994), of the eight staff members who had been asked by family members if they could be present, one was refused the request. Chalk (1995) undertook a similar, but larger, survey ($n = 50$), where 24 respondents had experience of relatives witnessing resuscitation. Interestingly, only 18 would allow relatives to be present in the future. Whilst this is the majority, it is well worth considering the views of the six who would no longer encourage relatives into the resuscitation room – clearly, 25% is an important figure, and further exploration of this group's view would have been a positive endeavour in seeking a balanced perspective. Whilst 67% believed families should have the choice to be with the patient if accompanied by a practitioner, only 21% would actually offer the invitation – presumably the remaining 79% would wait for the relative to formally ask to be present. In a European study undertaken by Fulbrook *et al.* (2005), 35 nurses (28%; of whom 22 were from the UK) had been approached by a family member requesting to be present during resuscitation. Of this subset of 35, only seven nurses (two from the UK and five from the rest of Europe) reported that they had a unit protocol that covered family presence during resuscitation.

Recent guidelines (as detailed above) suggest that relatives have a right to witness the resuscitation attempt and should be invited to do so; however, this needs to be balanced with current resources and perceived benefit to the patient (Fulbrook *et al.*, 2007). What is essential is that each unit develops its own workable guidelines for witnessing resuscitation; these guidelines should consider the frequency of the event, the resources available to manage the process, the debriefing process for staff and the relative and how ongoing professional counselling services (considered advisable) could be offered to the witnessing relative(s).

The role of the designated healthcare professional responsible for supporting witnessing relatives is to:

- Brief them about what to expect prior to entering the resuscitation area – family members should be warned that on occasions they may be asked to leave, for example for the purpose of obtaining radiographs or to avoid obstructing the work of the resuscitation team.
- Provide a running commentary with appropriate explanations.
- Help the relatives to communicate their presence to the patient.
- Respond truthfully and realistically to questions.
- Maintain a safe environment.
- Assess continually the relatives' emotional and physical status.
- Accompany (if possible) the family members if they wish to leave the scene, continuing to liaise with the resuscitation team on their behalf.
- Provide an opportunity for relatives to reflect on the resuscitation process after the event, participate in resuscitation team debriefing, providing feedback with respect to the needs and concerns expressed by them.

(Resuscitation Council UK, 1996; RCN, 2004;
Baskett *et al.*, 2005; Fulbrook *et al.*, 2007)

The decision of a family member about whether or not to be present during resuscitation of a relative should be made freely by the family member, without coercion or pressure. Barratt & Wallis (1998) examined the views of 35 recently bereaved family members about whether they would have liked to have been offered the opportunity to witness resuscitation of their relative. Of these, 15 wanted to have this option.

In a more recent study that explored the attitudes of 55 relatives about whether they should be present during resuscitation, 47% responded that they would wish to be with their relative even in such situations (Grice *et al.*, 2003). As the public becomes more accustomed to witnessing such scenes on television, the progression of them wanting to be close to their own relatives at such critical times is easy to rationalise. Clearly, people are generally more informed and knowledgeable about what happens during resuscitation; as such it becomes questionable whether healthcare professionals should exclude them from the process. This becomes even more difficult to justify for the relative who may have commenced CPR in the home and/or witnessed it in the back of the ambulance (Adams, 1994; van der Woning, 1999).

Interestingly, in the study undertaken at the Foote Hospital, 100% of the witnessing relatives believed that the healthcare team had done everything possible for their loved one; this will clearly have a positive impact in the early stages of their grief management (Hanson & Strawser, 1992).

PERCEIVED ADVANTAGES AND DISADVANTAGES OF RELATIVES WITNESSING RESUSCITATION

Similar themes of practitioners' perceptions of the advantages and disadvantages of family presence recur throughout the literature. Practitioners often focus on the potential disadvantages, many of which are not substantiated by research; however, it has to be borne in mind that the majority of current research studies surrounding relatives witnessing resuscitation are limited. Box 6.1 summarises the perceived advantages and disadvantages of witnessing resuscitation. It is worth noting that it has been reported that practitioners initially opposing family presence have striking shifts in opinion when their experiences with family presence do not confirm their concerns and the benefits to families become apparent (McGayhey, 2002).

CONCLUSION

It is almost inevitable that the concept of witnessing resuscitation will remain in the public forum and, as such, very likely that

Box 6.1 Perceived advantages and disadvantages of relatives witnessing resuscitation

Advantages

- Bonding between patients, patients' family members and caregivers is facilitated.
- Family members can observe the efforts of the healthcare team.
- Family members can provide comfort to their loved one and speak words of encouragement.
- Family's freedom to obtain closure; acceptance of outcome is facilitated.
- Family members can touch the patient while the patient is still warm.
- Staff may view the patient as part of a loving family, recognising individuality.
- The mystery of activities behind the closed doors of resuscitation room is reduced.
- Being present during the resuscitation, rather than hearing only a verbal account, may dispel family members' doubts about the course of events – promoting the belief that everything possible was done.
- A holistic approach, with acknowledgement of family as part of the patient, is fostered.

Disadvantages

- Patients' family members may disrupt the resuscitation efforts; prior coping strategies are unknown.
- Healthcare staff may not be able to control their own emotions.
- Patients' families may be offended at sights and potentially engage in negative behaviour.
- Fear of litigation might inhibit staff from performing necessary tasks well.
- The potential exists for long-term emotional scarring, with violent, traumatic memories of the event.
- The long-term effects on family's emotional status are unknown.
- Stress for staff involved may be increased.

- Patients' confidentiality may be violated.
- Patients' consent is impossible to gain.
- Patients' families might not understand the tasks and procedures performed.
- Having the patient's family present might influence the decision about the duration of the resuscitation effort.
- Relatives may become distressed when the decision is made to abandon the resuscitation attempt.
- Relatives may have an unrealistic expectation of the success rate of resuscitation.
- Consumes the whole time of one staff member to facilitate the process.

practitioners working within a variety of healthcare settings will be approached by a relative requesting this option. Regardless of whether or not practitioners choose to endorse the concept of relatives witnessing resuscitation, it is sensible that collaborative policies are designed to guide and support the needs of staff in their practice, especially when dealing with distressed families who wish to be present. A structured and supportive approach has the potential to facilitate a positive beginning in the grieving process through the knowledge and belief that everything possible was done for their loved one.

REFERENCES

Adams S (1994) Should relatives be allowed to watch resuscitation? A sister's experience. *BMJ* **308**: 1687–1689.

American Heart Association in collaboration with the International Liaison Committee on Resuscitation (AHA and ILCOR) (2000) Guidelines for cardiopulmonary resuscitation and emergency cardiovascular care. *Circulation* **102**(suppl 8): 1–374.

Back D, Rooke V (1994) The presence of relatives in the resuscitation room. *Nurs Times* **90**(30): 34–35.

Barratt F, Wallis DN (1998) Relatives in the resuscitation room: Their point of view. *J Acc Emerg Med* **15**(2): 109–111.

Baskett PJF, Steen PA, Bossaert, L (2005) European Council Guidelines for Resuscitation 2005. Section 8. The ethics of resuscitation and end-of-life decisions. *Resuscitation* **67**(supp. 1): S171–S180.

Boyd R (2000) Witnessed resuscitation by relatives. *Resuscitation* **43**(3): 171–176.

Chalk A (1995) Should relatives be present in the resuscitation room? *Acc Emerg Nurs* **3**(2): 58–61.

Crisci C (1994) Local factors may influence decision (letter). *BMJ* **309**(6951): 406.

Department of Health (DH) (2001) *Reference Guide to Consent for Examination or Treatment, DH 23617*. Available at: http://www.dh.gov.uk/en/Publichealth/Scientificdevelopmentgeneticsandbioethics/Consent/index.htm (accessed 10 June 2009).

Doyle CJ, Post H, Burney RE, Maino J, Keefe M, Rhee KJ (1987) Family participation during resuscitation: An option. *Ann Emerg Med* **16**(6): 673–675.

Eichhorn DJ, Meyers TA, Guzzetta CE *et al* (2001) Family presence during invasive procedures and resuscitation: Hearing the voice of the patient. *Am J Nurs* **101**(5): 48–55.

Fein, JA, Ganesh J, Alpern ER (2004) Medical staff attitudes toward family presence during paediatric procedures. *Paediatr Emerg Care* **20**(4): 224–227.

Fulbrook P, Albarran, J, Latour JM (2005) A European survey of critical care nurses' attitudes and experiences of having family members present during cardiopulmonary resuscitation. *Intl J Nurs Stud* **42**(5): 557–568.

Fulbrook P, Latour, J, Albarran, J, *et al* (2007) The presence of family members during cardiopulmonary resuscitation: European Federation of Critical Care Nursing associations, European Society of Paediatric and Neonatal Intensive Care and European Society of Cardiology Council on Cardiovascular Nursing and Allied Professions Joint Position Statement. *Connect: World Crit Care Nurs* **5**(4): 86–88.

Gold KJ, Gorenflo DW, Thomas L, Schwenk TL, Bratton SL (2006) Physician experience with family during cardiopulmonary resuscitation in children. *Paediatr Crit Care Med* **7**(5): 428–433.

Goldstein A, Berry K, Callaghan A (1997) Resuscitation witnessed by relatives. *BMJ* **314**: 144.

Goldsworth JE (1998) Your patient is undergoing resuscitation. Where's the family? *Nursing* **28**: 52–53.

Grice AS, Picton P & Deakin CD (2003) Study examining attitudes of staff, patients and relatives to witnessed resuscitation in adult intensive care units. *Br J Anaesth* **91**(6): 820–824.

Hanson C, Strawser D (1992) Family presence during cardiopulmonary resuscitation: Foote Hospital emergency department's nine years perspective. *J Emerg Nurs* **18**(2): 104–106.

Mazer MA, Cox LA, Capon A (2006) The public's attitude and perception concerning witnessed cardiopulmonary resuscitation. *Crit Care Med* **34**(12): 2925–2928.

McGayhey PR (2002) Family presence during paediatric resuscitation: A focus on staff. *Crit Care Nurse* **22**(6): 29–34.

McLauchlan C (1997) Allowing relatives to witness resuscitation. *BMJ* **314**: 1044.

Meyers TA, Eichhorn DJ, Guzzetta CE (1998) Do families want to be present during CPR? A retrospective survey. *J Emerg Nurs* **24**: 400–405.

Osuagwu C (1991) ED codes: Keep the family out. *J Emerg Care* **17**(6): 363–364.

Royal College of Nursing (RCN) (2004) *Witnessing Resuscitation: Guidance for Nursing Staff*. RCN Publications, London.

Resuscitation Council UK (1996) *Should Relatives Witness Resuscitation? A Report from a Project Team of the Resuscitation Council UK*. Resuscitation Council UK, London.

Robinson SM, Mackenzie-Ross S, Campbell Hewson GL, Egleston CV, Prevost AT (1998) Psychological effect of witnessed resuscitation on bereaved relatives. *Lancet* **352**(9128): 614–617.

Stewart K, Bowker L (1997) Resuscitation witnessed by relatives might lead to a complaint for breach of confidentiality. *BMJ* **314**: 145.

Van der Woning M (1999) Relatives in the resuscitation area: A phenomenological study. *Nurs Crit Care* **4**(4): 186–192.

Walker WM (2006) Witnessed resuscitation: A concept analysis. *Int J Nurs Stud* **43**(3): 377–387.

Weslien M, Nilstun T, Lundqvist A, Fridlund B (2006) Narratives about resuscitation – Family members differ about presence. *Eur J Cardiovasc Nurs* **5**(1): 68–74.

7 | Organ Donation

Rachel Hodge and Liz Armstrong

INTRODUCTION

Transplants are one of the most miraculous achievements of modern medicine. Well over a million people worldwide have had their lives saved or their quality of life improved by an organ transplant. Many more will benefit from a tissue transplant. From modest beginnings, transplantation has rapidly reached the forefront of modern medicine, and the increasing effectiveness of transplantation means that many more patients can be considered for treatment in this way.

> 'We should rejoice that medicine, in its service of life, has found in transplantation a new way of serving the human family.'
>
> (John Paul II, 1991)

The aim of this chapter is to understand the process of organ donation.

LEARNING OUTCOMES

At the end of this chapter, the reader will be able to:

- ❏ Outline the background to organ donation.
- ❏ Outline discussions about organ donation with the patient's family.
- ❏ Discuss the role of the coroner in organ/tissue donation.
- ❏ Discuss initiatives to maximise organ donation in the future.
- ❏ Discuss brain stem death.
- ❏ Discuss The Human Tissue Act 2004 and organ donation.

BACKGROUND TO ORGAN DONATION

Transplants first began at the beginning of the 20th century (Box 7.1). Sir Magdi Yacoub has described transplantation as 'one of the great success stories of the latter half of the 20th century'

Box 7.1 Transplantation milestones (UK Transplant, 2007). Reproduced from www.nhsbt.nhs.uk with kind permission of the Organ Donation and Transplantation Directorate, NHS Blood and Transport

- 1902 Alexis Carrel demonstrates method of joining blood vessels to make organ transplant feasible.
- 1905 First reported cornea transplant takes place Olmutz, Moravia (now Czech Republic) in December 1905.
- 1918 Blood transfusion becomes established.
- 1948 Foundation of the National Health Service.
- 1954 First successful kidney transplant operation performed in Boston, USA.
- 1960 First UK living donor kidney transplant, performed at The Royal Infirmary, Edinburgh.
- 1963 First liver transplant in Denver, USA.
- 1965 First kidney transplant in UK using organ from a dead person.
- 1967 First heart transplant operation performed by Dr Christiaan Barnard in South Africa.
- 1968 First heart transplant in UK.
- 1968 First UK liver transplant, performed at Addenbrooke's Hospital, Cambridge.
- 1968 National Tissue Typing and Reference Laboratory (NTTRL) established at Southmead Hospital, Bristol.
- 1971 Kidney donor card introduced in the UK.
- 1972 National Organ Matching and Distribution Service (NOMDS) founded in Bristol.
- 1979 NTTRL and NOMDS merge to become UK Transplant Service.
- 1979 UK heart transplant programme begins.
- 1980s First transplant co-ordinators appointed.
- 1981 UK kidney donor card changed to multi-organ card, including kidneys, corneas, heart, liver and pancreas.
- 1983 UK liver transplant programme begins.
- 1983 Launch of the UK Cornea Transplant Service (CTS).
- 1983 First combined heart and lung transplant in the UK.
- 1985 Lungs added to the UK donor card.
- 1986 First lung-only transplant in the UK.
- 1986 Establishment of the Bristol Eye Bank.

Continued

- 1987 First 'domino' UK heart transplant, where a patient receiving a heart and lungs transplant donates their healthy heart to another.
- 1989 Establishment of the Manchester Eye Bank.
- 1991 UK Transplant Service becomes special health authority and is renamed United Kingdom Transplant Support Service Authority (UKTSSA).
- 1993 UKTSSA moves to purpose-built accommodation at Stoke Gifford, Bristol.
- 1994 NHS Organ Donor Register established.
- 1994 First living donor liver transplant in UK.
- 1995 First living donor lung lobe transplant in UK.
- 2000 UK Transplant takes over from UKTSSA with new, extended remit.
- 2001 First lung transplant from a non-heart beating donor.
- 2005 UK Transplant merges with National Blood Service to form NHS Blood and Transplant.
- 2005 First partial face transplant carried out in France on 27 November.
- 2006 Introduction of the Human Tissue Acts 2004 in England, Wales and Northern Ireland, and the Human Tissue (Scotland) Act 2006.

(UK Transplant, 2007). Some important milestones in the history of transplantation are listed in Box 7.1.

Success of transplants

Transplants are so successful that a year after surgery:

- 94% of kidneys in living donor transplants are functioning well.
- 88% of kidneys from people who have died are functioning well.
- 86% of liver transplants are functioning well.
- 84% of heart transplants are functioning well.
- 77% of lung transplants are functioning well.
- 73% of heart/lung transplants are functioning well.

In 2007:

- 3086 organ transplants were carried out, thanks to the generosity of 1495 donors.

- A total of 2137 patients received a kidney, pancreas or combined kidney/pancreas transplant.
- 949 lives were saved in the UK through a heart, lung, liver or combined heart/lung, liver/kidney, liver/pancreas or heart/kidney transplant.
- A further 2402 people had their sight restored through a cornea transplant.
- 14 201 229 people registered on the organ donor register at 31 March 2007.

(UK Transplant, 2007)

Demand for organs

Between April 2006 and March 2007, 3086 organ transplants were carried out in the UK (Figure 7.1). However, demand for organs and in some cases tissues, particularly corneas, can outstrip the supply of donated organs and tissues. With 7234 patients on the active transplant waiting list at the end of March 2007 (UK Transplant, 2007), the demand for organs is increasing rapidly. Too few human organs for transplantation, too many patients in need, and the gap widens (Figure 7.1) (Randall, 1991).

UK Donation and Transplant Waiting List

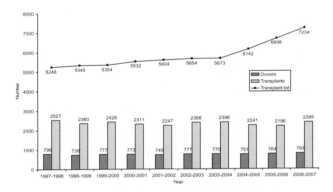

Fig 7.1 UK donation and transplant waiting list. Reproduced from www.nhsbt.nhs. uk with kind permission of the Organ Donation and Transplantation Directorate, NHS Blood and Transplant

Potential donors

A national potential donor audit of all deaths in 341 intensive care units (ICUs) in the UK over a recent 33-month-period revealed the potential to achieve a donation rate of 23.2 donors per million population, well above the current rate of 12.9 per million population (UK Transplant, 2006) (Figure 7.2).

Whilst factors influencing how many transplant operations take place are multifaceted, two overriding influences on the potential number of deceased donor organs that are available for donation are:

- The number of people who die in circumstances that facilitate donation.
- The willingness of the 'nominated' or 'qualifying person' (Human Tissue Act, 2004) to allow organ donation to proceed (UK Transplant, 2006).

Department of Health policy

The Department of Health's (DH) policy for the development of transplant services in England is set out in *Saving Lives, Valuing Donors, a Transplant Framework for England* (DH, 2003), which clearly outlines that the NHS can only meet the need of organs and tissues for transplant if:

- People are made aware of the possibilities of donating organs and tissues, and are willing to do so.
- The NHS identifies all potential donors.
- Organs and tissues donated are retrieved by skilled professionals and used effectively.

In this policy Rosie Winterton, Minister of State, stated 'organ and tissue donation is entirely dependent on the altruism of ordinary members of the public. Their generosity must be welcomed and appreciated. Their life-saving gift must be respected and received with gratitude' (DH, 2003)

CLASSIFICATION OF DONORS

The manner, time and place of death determine whether a person's organs are suitable for donation. Organ donors can be classified as either 'heart beating' or 'non-heart beating'.

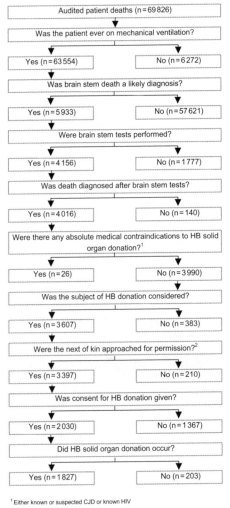

¹ Either known or suspected CJD or known HIV

² Includes cases where the next of kin made the approach

Fig 7.2 A breakdown from audited patient deaths to heart-beating donors. Reproduced from www.nhsbt.nhs.uk with kind permission of the Organ Donation and Transplantation Directorate, NHS Blood and Transplant. ¹Either known or suspected CJD or known HIV. ²Includes cases where the next of kin made the approach

Heart-beating organ donors

Most donated organs come from patients who are under 75 years of age, ventilated, are being cared for in the ICU and whose death has been certified by brain stem death (BSD) criteria. These patients' organs remain perfused with blood up to the point that they are removed and this means that families need to say their goodbyes whilst the patient remains on a ventilator and with a heartbeat. These patients are called 'heart-beating donors' and are able to donate heart, lungs, liver, kidneys, pancreas and bowel, as well as all tissues. Organs may be transplanted as single organ transplants or on occasions as multiple transplants such as heart and lung, liver and small bowel, and kidney and pancreas.

Non-heart beating organ donors

Organs can also be donated from patients who are under 65 years of age shortly after death following cardiorespiratory arrest. Death is certified at the time the heart stops – from this moment, organs are deprived of oxygen and begin to deteriorate rapidly. The opportunity to retrieve the organ is short; if organs are to be used, they have to be retrieved and transplanted quickly. It is usual that these patients are nursed in an ICU or critical care setting and a plan has been established to withdraw treatment based on the futility of the patient's situation. Organ donation can be facilitated if the patient dies shortly after withdrawal of treatment. These patients are called 'non-heart beating organ donors' and they are able to donate kidneys and in some cases liver and lungs, as well as all tissues.

Some families may be more comfortable with this type of donation as it fulfils social expectations of death, in that families can witness the last breath and cessation of heart beat – not an option if the deceased is a heart-beating donor.

Tissue donors

Many patients who die in hospital can donate tissues to help others (from the wards, ICUs, emergency departments, palliative care units and the community following cardiorespiratory death). Tissue donation means that someone else's life can be improved, or even saved, after the death of a loved one. Donation of tissues can allow relatives of patients to fulfil their loved ones' wishes to donate in the event of their death, and many bereaved families take comfort in the knowledge that their loved one has helped others in this way. Up to 50 patients can be helped as a result of tissue donation.

Tissues are retrieved in the mortuary following death, usually within 24 h (tissue does not deteriorate immediately following the cessation of the heartbeat because of its low metabolic requirements, allowing more time for tissue retrieval). Tissues are matched according to age and size, rather than blood group; tissue recipients do not need to take anti-rejection drugs. However, early identification and referral of potential tissue donors is crucial in ensuring that the quality of the tissues retrieved is optimised.

Eye donation

Patients aged from 3 years upwards can donate eyes for transplant. There is no upper age limit for eye donation.

When the eyes are donated, both the corneas and sclera can be used for transplantation.

In order for both corneal and sclera donation to proceed, the whole eye is retrieved by specially trained personnel. Families may be concerned that their loved one will look different after eye retrieval. Reassurance can be given to the families of eye donors that they will still be able to view their loved one following eye donation, although they need to be supported as there may be some puffiness, blueing and discolouration following the retrieval.

Skin donation

Patients aged 17 years upwards can donate skin for transplant. There is no upper age limit for skin donation.

Skin is retrieved from the back of the body and the legs. Donated skin is not full thickness; it is only tissue-paper thin.

Donated skin is used to treat major burns and acts as a temporary protective dressing. It can save lives by stopping infections, stimulating underlying tissues and preparing a good dermal bed for later skin grafting.

Heart valve donation

Patients from 32 weeks gestation to 65 years of age can donate heart valves.

Aortic and pulmonary valves and patches of the pulmonary artery are dissected at specialist heart valve banks following the retrieval of the entire heart. Following heart retrieval the chest is closed.

Donated heart valves are used in both adults and children with diseased or damaged heart valves. Heart valve patches are generally used in patients with congenital heart problems, many of whom are young children.

Bone and meniscus donation

Patients from 17 years of age upwards can donate bone for transplant. There is no upper age limit for bone donation. Patients below the age of 50 years of age can also donate meniscus.

Bone can be donated from the hip to just below the knee. The donated bone is replaced with a specifically designed prosthesis, after which the leg is fully reconstructed. One donation can provide bone to help up to 30 different patients and can be used in types of orthopaedic surgery such as:

- Revision joint placement.
- Spinal fusion.
- Major bone replacement.

Meniscus can be removed from within the knee joint as part of the bone retrieval and used to repair injured knee joints.

Tendons

Patients between the ages of 17 and 60 years can donate tendons for transplant.

The Achilles and patella tendons can be used to repair the anterior and posterior cruciate ligaments in the knee joint and are therefore used primarily for sports injuries.

Blood vessels

Patients between the ages of 17 and 50 years can donate blood vessels for transplant.

Blood vessels can be retrieved and used in patients who have vascular problems. If families who consent to blood vessel donation also consent to heart valve and bone donation, the same incisions made for bone and heart valve donation can be utilised for blood vessel retrieval.

IDENTIFICATION AND REFERRAL OF TISSUE DONORS

The families of all potential tissue donors should be offered the option of tissue donation. Twenty four per cent of the population have registered their wish to donate in the event of their death and therefore the organ donor register should be checked when a patient dies in hospital. Even if the patient is not on the organ donation register, families should still be offered the option of tissue donation as many people carry donor cards or have expressed a wish in their lifetime to donate in the event of their death.

For information and support, staff should contact the donor transplant co-ordinator (DTC).

General criteria for organ donation

The general criteria for organ donation include:

- Catastrophic and irreversible neurological injury leading to BSD.
- The patient's condition is such that continuing critical care is considered futile, and withdrawal of treatment is being considered.

There are no absolute age restrictions, although solid organs are rarely taken from patients over 80 years of age. Specific criteria might apply in non-heart beating donation; the DTC would give further advice.

There are few absolute contraindications for organ donation, e.g. certain cancers or a confirmed diagnosis of human immuno-deficiency virus (HIV) or known or suspected classical or variant Creutzfeldt–Jacob disease (CJD). Even patients with known transmissible conditions may be able to donate if there is a recipient for whom benefits exceed risks. The Advisory Committee on the Microbiological Safety of Blood and Tissues for Transplantation (MSBT) provides national guidance on donor evaluation and testing (DH, 2000). The guidance is updated on the website and the DTC will be aware of the latest advice and guidance.

DONATION/RETRIEVAL PROCEDURE

This is a cooperative effort between several visiting surgical teams and the staff from the donating hospital. An anaesthetist accompanies heart-beating donors to theatre and continues management of ventilation. All organ donors continue to be cared for with the utmost respect and dignity afforded to every patient undergoing a surgical procedure. Organs are perfused, then removed and packed in ice and transported to their destination. Last offices are then performed.

Role of the donor transplant co-ordinator

When it has been established that a patient could be an organ donor it is essential that the on-call DTC is informed so that the donation can be conducted in a timely fashion. The hospital switchboard will be able to do this.

The DTC plays an important supportive role for all healthcare professionals, particularly those working in the critical care areas, and for the families of potential organ and tissue donors. The DTC can offer expert advice and guidance on the concept of the diagnosis of death by brain stem testing, the criteria for suitability for donation and the management of the donor in critical care (Box 7.2).

Discussions about organ donation with the patient's family

Some medical and nursing staff may find it difficult to ask the patient's family to consider the option of organ/tissue donation for transplantation. The DTC will be able to support healthcare teams in doing this.

The healthcare staff caring for the patient, together with the DTC, can meet the family after it has been established that the family understands and accepts the patient's BSD or that the patient's continued treatment is futile and withdrawal of treatment is planned.

Empirical evidence suggests that having a DTC present during the donation approach is linked with lower refusal rates from

---

> **Box 7.2 Donor family memories (UK Transplant, 2008).**
> **Reproduced from http://www.nhsbt.nhs.uk with kind**
> **permission of the Organ Donation and Transplantation**
> **Directorate, NHS Blood and Transport**
>
> Little Jade Stoner loved making people happy. The pretty
> Dorset schoolgirl was never seen without a smile and always
> wanted to help others, especially when they were sad. On 24
> September 2006, whilst playing on her bike outside her family
> home, the seven-year-old was hit by a car. Hours later, doctors
> at Bournemouth's Royal Hospital told her parents she would
> never recover. 'That's when we knew what Jade would have
> wanted,' said mum Debbie, 'she would have wanted to donate
> her organs.'
>
> Sikh Jagmohan Taank fulfilled his Gurus' teachings when he
> donated his organs for transplant to help others after his death.
> The thoughtful six-foot tall 'gentle giant' made the final decision
> to donate much easier for his family by carrying a donor card
> – and letting them know of his wish to donate organs before
> his tragic death. Jagmohan, known as 'Monna' to his family,
> was a fit, 26-year-old security officer when he complained of a
> severe headache, collapsed and was rushed to an ICU in
> Coventry, West Midlands, in August 2002.

family members, potentially as a result of what that individual
can bring to the discussion in relation to specialist knowledge
(Klieger *et al.*, 1994; Shafer *et al.*, 2004).

Ethical principles
To ensure that the highest ethical practice is maintained when
approaching families for organ donation, the following principles
are recommended:

- *Respect:* Treating the person who has died/who is dying with
  respect at all times.
- *Understanding:* Realising that to many families their love and
  feelings towards the person who has died are as strong as they
  were in life.

- *Consent/lack of objection:* Ensuring that consent/lack of objection is sought and given on the basis that a person is fully exercising informed choice.
- *Time and space:* Recognising that families may need time to consider whether to agree with donation and will not want to feel under pressure to agree.
- *Skill and sensitivity:* Staff need to be sensitive to the needs of the families of patients who have died and sufficient staff skilled in bereavement care should be available.
- *Cultural competence:* Attitudes to organ donation, and particularly to the use of organs and tissues after death, differ between religions and cultural groups; healthcare staff need to be aware of these factors and respond to them with sensitivity.
- *A gift relationship:* The recognition that tissue or organs are given as a gift to help others, and so deserve gratitude.

(Gortmaker *et al.*, 1998)

Responsibilities of the DTC during the discussion with the family include:

- *Establishing consent for organ donation:* If the patient's wishes have already been established by checking the Organ Donor Register (see the section on The Human Tissue Act 2004 (HTA) and organ donation), the family need to be informed of this. If the wishes of the patient are not known then the DTC establishes consent from the family. The family may stipulate what organs/tissues may or may not be removed but conditions relating to the potential recipients are not acceptable.
- *Establishing family wishes regarding the disposal of any organs/ tissue taken which do not get transplanted:* Research options and/ or lawful disposal are discussed with the family.
- *Taking a history:* Establishing whether any medical, social or behavioural risk factors exist by completing a detailed history about the potential donor.
- *Discussing with the family the timings of the donation procedure.*
- *Reassuring the family regarding visiting opportunities:* Advising that they will have the opportunity to visit the deceased after donation.
- *Ascertaining any specific requirements for last offices:* Some families will wish to assist in the final care or may wish certain

items remain with their loved one. The DTC could take hand-prints and locks of hair for the family if that is something that they would like.

- *Providing follow-up care:* Thanking the family for their time and ensuring they have the DTC's contact details, details about recipients of the donated organs and where appropriate letters/cards which may be sent from the organ recipients will be forwarded to the family.
- *Providing follow-up on the recipient's progress:* As and when the donor family want it.

Following the family interview, the DTC continues the donation process. This involves caring for the donor, which is always consistent with optimal patient care. By managing the donor carefully at this stage, we can hope to improve the chances of survival in the transplant patient.

Using blood group compatibility, organs such as the heart, lungs and liver are matched with patients waiting for transplant in the UK and Ireland. Kidneys are matched later using HLA (human leukocyte antigens) tissue type match criteria.

Surgical teams are mobilised from the transplanting hospitals to the donor hospital and the donor is taken to theatre for the retrieval to begin.

Role of the coroner in organ/tissue donation

Coroners cannot give consent for organ/tissue donation but can agree to organ/tissue donation proceeding if they believe that donation will not interfere with their legal responsibilities to establish the cause of death. In most circumstances, the coroner will be able to allow organ/tissue donation to proceed if presented with all the relevant information and steps are taken to preserve possible evidence. The coroner may ask the transplant retrieval surgeons to take further safeguards for the judicial process. These may include:

- Making notes and taking photographs of external injuries.
- Collecting blood and urine samples.
- Supplying detailed summaries of the retrieval operation.
- Having a Home Office pathologist present during retrieval.

INITIATIVES TO MAXIMISE ORGAN DONATION IN THE FUTURE

One of the most significant developments in focusing on the discrepancy between organ demand and supply was the initiative by UK Transplant to assess the actual levels of potential organ donors by auditing every patient death from deaths which occur in every ICU. This national potential donor audit commenced in January 2003. The results of the audit indicate a relatives refusal rate for organ donation at 40% for deceased heart-beating donation, 46% for deceased non-heart beating donation and 70% for 'non white' groups (UK Transplant, 2006). Initiatives to increase consent for organ donation are based on these results.

Organ Donation Task Force

The Organ Donation Task Force was established in 2006 to identify obstacles to donation and to suggest solutions to increase the number of transplants. Three barriers to donation were identified:

- Donor identification and referral.
- Donor co-ordination.
- Organ retrieval arrangements.

Matters needing attention across the three categories included:

- Legal and ethical issues.
- The role of the NHS.
- Organisation of co-ordination and retrieval.
- Training.
- Public recognition and public promotion of donation.

In 2008, the 14 recommendations suggested by the task force were accepted in their entirety. It is envisaged that once implemented there will be a 50% increase in donors by 2012, equating to an extra 1200 transplants per year (700 kidney transplants). More information is available at www.uktransplant.org.uk.

Embedded donor transplant co-ordinators

As part of the ODTF recommendations, DTCs will be embedded in all hospitals with a potential for organ donation. It has been shown that having a specifically–trained, knowledgeable, family-focused, motivated health professional who has the time to discuss all aspects of the organ donation decision-making process with family members is linked to increased consent rates for organ donation (Gortmaker *et al.*, 1998; UK Transplant, 2006).

Collaborative approach/requesting

This is where the approach/request for organ donation is done by the clinician caring for the patient and the DTC together. Empirical evidence suggests that having a DTC present during the donation approach is linked with lower refusal rates from family members, potentially as a result of what that individual can bring to the discussion in relation to specialist knowledge (Kleiger *et al.*, 1994; Shafer *et al.*, 2004). These findings underpin the need for a skilled, well-informed, motivated individual, who has time to spend with the family, in early discussions about organ donation.

The ACRE (Assessment of Collaborative Requesting) was a pragmatic, multi-centre, prospective, open, randomised controlled trial that was carried out throughout critical care units in the UK. Its aims were to compare whether relatives of brain stem dead patients are more likely to consent to organ donation when interviewed by the clinical team alone or when interviewed by the clinical team and the DTC. This trial, which is now complete, may have wide-ranging implications for future policy and procedure regarding the approach and discussion about organ donation.

Non-heart beating organ donation

This is where patients donate organs after cardiac death. The transplant retrieval surgeons are in theatre when treatment is withdrawn on a patient where the decision has been made that continued active life support is no longer in the patient's interest. Non-heart beating organ donation was the norm before the introduction of BSD tests. An argument supporting non-heart beating organ donation is that some family members struggle with the diagnosis of BSD, and might believe that the patients are not dead as their heart is still beating, their chest is still moving and they look alive (Long, 2007).

Increasing the number of people registering their wishes on the organ donor register

There is a belief that family members will agree to organ donation if their deceased relatives stated in life that they wanted to donate. Now that the UK has legislation to prioritise consent given in life regarding organ donation over the wishes of the family, there is an increase in publicity to encourage people to register their wishes and maybe in the future we will see a change from 'requesting' organ donation to 'informing' about organ donation. The wording publicity material may be changed to:

Already carry a card?

Carrying the card is a great start, but to be a registered organ donor you need to *join the NHS Organ Donor Register* at www.organdonation.nhs.

BRAIN STEM DEATH

Most people believe that death occurs when a person's heart beat and breathing stop. However, as cardiopulmonary function can now be maintained by artificial means, death cannot always be equated with cessation of spontaneous heart beat. It is therefore important that healthcare professionals caring for patients, particularly in the critical care environment and emergency department setting, understand the concept of BSD and also the consequences of the declaration of BSD in order to support relatives of patients who are diagnosed as BSD.

Brain stem death was formally introduced in 1976 and has been ratified by the DH and medical royal colleges on several occasions since, most recently in October 2008. Its equation with human death is based on the concept that death entails the irreversible loss of those essential characteristics which are necessary to the existence of a living human person and, thus, the definition of death should be regarded as, 'The irreversible loss for consciousness, combined with the irreversible loss of the capacity to breathe' (Academy of the Medical Royal Colleges, 2008).

Causes of brain stem death

The brain stem comprises the medulla, pons and mesencephalon, and functions as a conduction pathway for motor and sensory impulses. The reticular formation is the central core of the brain stem and contains the vital centres responsible for respiration and cardiac activity.

The skull is a rigid compartment containing three components: brain tissue, arterial and venous blood, and cerebrospinal fluid (CSF). If there is an increase in the relative volume of one of these components, the volume of one or both of the other components must decrease – this is known as the Monroe–Kellie doctrine.

When intercranial pressure continues to rise, the contents of the cranial vault expand to a space of least resistence. This path within the skull is down towards the brain stem through the foramen magnum and is known as 'coning'. If this continues, the brain stem will be irreversibly destroyed.

Diagnosis of brain stem death

The clinical diagnosis of BSD in the UK relies on demonstrating the absence of brain stem reflexes.

Brain stem death is diagnosed by two independent doctors (one should be a consultant), neither of whom should be members of the transplant team. Two full sets of BSD tests should be performed.

Preconditions for testing include:

- The patient's condition is due to irreversible brain damage of known aetiology.
- The patient is deeply comatose, unresponsive and apnoeic with his/her lungs being artificially ventilated.
- No evidence that the coma is due to depressant drugs.
- No evidence that the coma is caused by hypothermia (greater than 34 °C)
- All circulatory, metabolic and endocrine disturbances must have been excluded.
- All potentially reversible causes of apnoea (presence of muscle relaxants and high spinal injury) must have been excluded.
- The patient is cardiovascular-optimised.

Tests for brain stem death

- The pupils are fixed and do not respond to sharp changes in the intensity of light.

- No corneal reflex when a piece of cotton wool is drawn over the exposed cornea.
- The oculo-vestibular reflexes are absent when ice-cold water is injected into the patient's ear.
- No motor response within the cranial nerve distribution can be elicited by adequate stimulation of any somatic area (supraorbital pressure).
- No cough reflex to bronchial stimulation.
- No respiratory response to hypercarbia.

Test: 100% oxygen therapy is delivered through the ventilator for 15 min prior to disconnection to ensure that the patient will not become hypoxic or is adversely affected by the test. The patient is then disconnected from the ventilator and their carbon dioxide is allowed to rise to 6.65 kPa.

Brain death diagnosis in young children and infants
A report of the working party of the British Paediatric Association of 1991 suggested that 'for children over the age of two months, the criteria used to establish death should be the same as adults. Between 37 weeks of gestation and two months of age, it is rarely possible confidently to diagnose death as a result of cessation of brain stem reflexes, and below 37 weeks' gestation this criteria can not be applied'.

HUMAN TISSUE ACT (2004) AND ORGAN DONATION
The revised Human Tissue Act 2004 (HTA) evolved in response to the organ retention scandals of the 1990s. Whilst Alder Hey and Bristol Royal Infirmary remain in the public mind when storage of organs without consent is discussed, the practice was widespread. In 2001 Liam Donaldson, the Chief Medical Officer, revealed that more than 100 000 examples of organs and tissues being stored without consent could be found in hospitals and medical schools throughout the UK (BBC, 2001).

The Human Tissue Authority has overseen the HTA from its inception and continues to license a number of activities and inspects to ensure compliance with the Act and licence conditions. The Human Tissue Authority will have a general role in informing the public and the Secretary of State about issues within its remit including:

- Storage and use of human bodies and tissue, and removal of tissue from human bodies, for scheduled purposes.
- Importing/exporting of bodies and human tissue for scheduled purposes.
- Disposal of human tissue, including imported tissue, following its use in medical treatment or for scheduled purposes.

The overarching principle of the HTA is that without valid and appropriate consent, it is illegal for organs or tissues to be removed, stored or utilised for any purpose. The Act has far-reaching powers, with cadaveric organ donation being a small part of the whole, as the Act also encompasses removal of material from the living. The majority of the information related to organs and tissue donation is covered by Code of Practice 2.

The HTA has had an impact on the work of DTCs, primarily in relation to the consent procedure. The aim of the HTA is to make the wishes and choices of the deceased paramount. Therefore, if any competent person has registered on the organ donor register (ODR) or carries an organ donor card this can be deemed as valid consent. Consequently, it is lawful to proceed with retrieval of organs regardless of whether the family concurs with this choice.

However, although this seeks to honour the wishes of the deceased, it is not without difficulties. The Act gives support to the ODR as consent for removal of organs and tissues but it does not include storage, research or the removal of blood for the tests required to permit transplantation. Consequently, by refusal to give consent at this stage, the wishes of the deceased can be overridden (Box 7.3).

Box 7.3 Appropriate consent for deceased adult

- His/her consent before death.
- If no prior consent, consent of a nominated representative.
- If no representative, the consent of a qualifying relative.

The role of the DTC is to facilitate the wishes of the deceased, whilst respecting the grief of their families. The DTC will aim to seek the opinions and fears of families about organ donation. The use of the ODR can help ease the discussion about organ donation. However, it must be remembered that as there is an opt-in system in the UK, not being registered does not preclude the donation request.

Any healthcare professional can access the ODR to see if a potential donor is registered. However, the DTC can ascertain the exact stated organs and tissues that the donor has consented to on the ODR. This is important, as when speaking to families one cannot ask about that which has not been consented to by the deceased. However, if the family offer, that is acceptable, and it is important that any approach is made in accordance with the Act.

When gaining consent from families, the HTA sets down a hierarchy of relationships. This is especially important when there is no ODR consent, but is also adhered to when gaining consent for storage or research when the potential donor is on the ODR. Firstly, any nominated representative must be sought; if there is no such person then consent should be gained by the highest-ranking relative. The next of kin (Box 7.4) could devolve the decision-making but the DTC should try to ascertain that there is no coercion.

Box 7.4 Hierarchy of qualifying relationships for the next of kin

- Spouse or partner.
- Parent or child.
- Brother or sister.
- Grandparent or grandchild.
- Child of a brother or sister.
- Stepfather or stepmother.
- Half brother or half sister.
- Longstanding friend.

Where there is more than one person of the same rank in the hierarchy, brother or sister for example, the consent of any one of them will make it lawful (not obligatory) to store or use tissue for a scheduled purpose.

The Human Tissue Act for Scotland was developed slightly after the initial act and has variations with regard to consent and the hierarchy of relatives. This can be viewed alongside the UK Act and the Codes of Practice at www.HTA.gov.uk.

CONCLUSION

This chapter has provided an understanding of the process of organ donation. The background to organ donation has been described, together with discussions about it with the patient's family. Initiatives to maximise organ donation in the future have been outlined. Important issues associated with BSD and the HTA (2004) have been discussed.

REFERENCES

Academy of the Medical Royal Colleges (2008) *A code of practice for the diagnosis and confirmation of death. Available at www.aomrc.org.uk/aomrc/ admin/reports/docs/DofD-final.pdf (accessed 26 November 2008).*

BBC (2001) Available at www.news.bbc.co.uk/1/hi/health/1144368.stm (accessed 26 November 2008).

Conference of Medical Royal Colleges and their Faculties in the United Kingdom (1991) *Diagnosis of Brain-Stem Death in Infants and Children.* British Paediatric Association, London. Available at www.aomrc. org.uk/aomrc/admin/reports/docs/section1DraftforConsultation 14.05.06.pdf (accessed 26 November 2008).

Department of Health (DH) (2000) *Guidance on the Microbiological Safety of Human Organs, Tissue and Cells used for Transplantation.* Department of Health, London. Available at www.doh.gov.uk/MSBT (accessed 26 November 2008).

Department of Health (DH) (2003) *Saving Lives, Valuing Donors, A Transplant Framework for England.* Department of Health, London.

Gortmaker S, Beasley C, Sheehy E, Lucas BA, Brigham LE, Grenvik A (1998) Improving the request process to increase family consent for organ donation. *J Transplant Coord* **4:** 210–217.

Human Tissue Act (2004) London. Available at www.legislation.hmso. gov/acts/acts20040030.htm (accessed 24 November 2007).

John Paul II (1991) *Address to the Participants of the Society for Organ Sharing,* 20 June 1991, Rome.

Klieger J, Nelson K, Davies R, *et al.* (1994) Analysis of factors influencing organ donation consent rates. *J Transplant* **4:** 132–134.

Long T (2007) *Brain-based criteria for diagnosing death: What does it mean to families approached about organ donation?* PhD Thesis, University of Southampton, Southampton. UK.

Randall T (1991) Too few human organs for transplantation, too many in need … and the gap widens. *JAMA*, **265**: 1223–1227.

Shafer TJ, Ehrle RN, Davies KD, *et al.* (2004) Increasing organ recovery from level 1 trauma centres: the in-house coordinator intervention. *Prog Transplant* **14**(3): 250–263.

UK Transplant (2006) *Potential Donor Audit: 36-month summary report 1st April 2003–31st March 2006.* Available at www.uktransplant.org.uk (accessed 24 November 2007).

UK Transplant (2007) Success rates. Available at www.uktransplant.org.uk (accessed 26 November 2008).

Breaking Bad News

8

Dan Higgins

INTRODUCTION

Bad news is any information that changes a person's view of the future in a negative way (Buckman, 1984). The concept of bad news is highly individualised and can be influenced by many factors, including social and cultural factors, age and religion. It is generally accepted that receiving news about deteriorating health, an incurable illness or death of a loved one is a negative experience.

The aim of this chapter is to understand the principles of breaking bad news.

LEARNING OUTCOMES

At the end of this chapter, the reader will be able to:

❑ Discuss the historical perspective to breaking bad news.
❑ List the objectives of breaking bad news.
❑ Outline effective communication skills.
❑ Explore barriers to breaking bad news effectively.
❑ Describe a systematic approach to breaking bad news.
❑ Explore the responses to grief and those receiving bad news.
❑ Discuss breaking bad news following an unexpected death.

HISTORICAL PERSPECTIVE TO BREAKING BAD NEWS

Traditionally, the role of breaking bad news has fallen to physicians, despite medical education only providing sparse formal preparation for this task (Vandekieft, 2001). However, it is now considered that breaking bad news should be undertaken by the most appropriate person, which may not necessarily be a doctor (Resuscitation Council UK, 2006). In some situations it will be more appropriate for a nurse to do it.

Historically, patients have been provided with very little information about their illness/disease process (Holland, 1989), possibly because many physicians considered receiving bad news as detrimental to the patients' treatment (Baile *et al.*, 2000). This practice has evolved over the last few decades, not only through advances in the management of cancer but also through patients' need for choice and requirements for information for which the Internet has been a catalyst. Honest disclosure of diagnoses, prognoses and treatment options allows patients to make informed healthcare decisions that are consistent with their goals and values (Mueller, 2002). Patients now see themselves, quite rightly, at the centre of their care and expect to have no information withheld from them.

Whilst breaking bad news is still part of a physician's work, thankfully now, supported by more education and training, it is common for other healthcare practitioners, particularly nurses, to undertake this vital role. This is perhaps inevitable, as nurses spend considerably more time communicating with patients, developing a relationship and a rapport.

Nurses should be well-equipped educationally to break bad news, as communication skills are a core component of nurse education. However, in some situations some may feel inexperienced to break bad news and be fearful of trespassing into what they perceive as another's role.

The patients' and relatives' responses to bad news are an ongoing process; thus if bad news has been broken by another discipline, the nurse is in an ideal position to assist the grieving process, to respond to their needs and answer questions. As a result nurses must develop skills in dealing with these situations.

The process of breaking bad news is not a sole responsibility of one professional group but is a shared responsibility, and assisting patients and their relatives to come to terms with the 'bad news' is the goal of a multidisciplinary team.

Breaking bad news will occur frequently in all clinical specialties, but certain areas such as critical care and oncology deal with bad news on a daily basis, thus there can be many opportunities for practitioners to develop skills and gain experience in these areas.

To measure effectiveness in delivering bad news is problematic and subjective. Research in this field is understandably lacking, although a wide variety of empirical studies document that physician–patient communication is suboptimal (Back *et al.*, 2005) Studies have consistently shown that the way a doctor or other health or social care professional delivers bad news places an indelible mark on the doctor/professional–patient relationship (Department of Health, Social Services & Public Safety (DHSSPS), 2000). The complexity associated with breaking bad news can create serious miscommunication, such as the recipient mis-understanding the prognosis of the illness or purpose of care (DHSSPS, 2000); it can also lead to dissatisfaction with care and potential complaints. There is evidence that giving bad news appropriately may facilitate coping and help identify which sources of support will help the recipient and his or her family (Hall, 2005); for these reasons alone the process of breaking bad news requires ongoing improvement.

OBJECTIVES OF BREAKING BAD NEWS
The key objectives when breaking bad news are to:

- Gather information.
- Relay information based on this at a pace appropriate to the recipient.
- Provide support for the recipient.
- Develop a strategy/management plan for the future.

This should be done in an environment where recipients feel supported, free to express themselves and have the opportunity to ask any questions.

The key to achieving these objectives is excellence in communication skills.

EFFECTIVE COMMUNICATION SKILLS
Breaking bad news is a complex communication task that requires expert verbal and non-verbal skills. The aspects of communication most valued by patients are those that help them and their families feel guided, build trust and support hope. While these may be abstract qualities, they follow from a concrete set of

communication skills that can be effectively taught and learned (Back *et al.*, 2005).

The essential components to effective communication when breaking bad news are:

- Listening.
- Questioning.
- Answering questions.
- Ascertaining.
- Responding appropriately to patients' and relatives' emotions.

Listening

Information is required from the recipient in order to pace the information that is to be delivered appropriately and at a level appropriate to that person's education and understanding. This process may identify how prepared the recipient is to receive the news, as in some cases the bad news may be expected. It is important that the practitioner looks prepared to listen, by sitting down, looking relaxed and not constrained by time. Eye contact should be maintained; to do otherwise may give the impression of a lack of interest.

Questioning

Closed and open-ended questions will be required. Closed questions are useful for collecting demographic data; open questions can help determine what the recipient wants to know, what he or she already knows and what is worrying him or her most (Brixey, 2004). Many recipients digress from the subject when answering questions, and this may be an avoidance strategy on their behalf and could indicate underlying emotions such as guilt. The practitioner may need to direct the discussion 'back on track', although this should be done diplomatically.

Answering questions

The recipient may also have many questions, which need answering honestly; certain points may need clarification. Medical terminology and jargon should be avoided at all times.

Ascertaining

Clarification and reiteration of issues may be required to ensure understanding of what the recipient has said and to ensure that he or she has understood what the practitioner has said.

Responding appropriately to patients' and relatives' emotions

Touch where appropriate; this may be in the form of holding hands or 'putting an arm around an individual' or 'providing a shoulder'. Allow patients and relatives time to express themselves and provide reassurance that the emotions the patient experiences are natural. For example, 'I know you must be very angry but… .'

Be observant, through observing body language for any underlying emotions, such as guilt. Showing empathy, exploring the recipient's understanding and acceptance of what he or she has just learned, and validating any expressed feelings can provide much-needed support (Buckman, 2005).

Communication traits to avoid

Lecturing

Lecturing occurs when the recipient is bombarded with large amounts of medical information; he or she rarely can digest and internalise the information, and confusion could ensue.

Blocking

This is where a recipient raises a question or point, and answering that question is avoided by the practitioner by redirecting the question. This represents a failure to address the recipient's predominant concerns. For example:

Patient: How will my children cope without me?
Nurse: I am sure they will be fine, now, how is your pain?

or

Patient: Doctor, how long do you think I have to live?
Doctor: I wouldn't worry about that right now, how are you getting on with the new drug?

Collusion

Collusion is where, because a recipient does not ask a certain question (because he or she does not wish to know such information), a practitioner does not raise a salient point. The practitioner may be subconsciously relieved that the question is not asked, thus avoiding the sensitive subject.

The patient or relative may think, 'If the doctor or nurse hasn't told me, it is not important'. For example, if a patient does not ask 'How long do you think I have to live?' that information is not relayed and discussion moves on to planned treatment, etc. Collusion means that difficult conversations about prognosis, cure and end of life do not occur.

BARRIERS TO BREAKING BAD NEWS

Upsetting situations

Breaking bad news to patients and relatives is not a pleasant task and one which many practitioners find stressful and upsetting; there are many reasons for this. It may be because of the practitioner's lack of confidence in dealing with distressed individuals and difficulty in empathising with that individual. Training in breaking bad news is only recently becoming emphasised in nursing and particularly medical education.

Coping with the grief response

Practitioners may also struggle to deal with anger and blame, which may be presented as a response to hearing bad news, particularly if that anger and blame is aimed personally or at the healthcare service. This may be combined with feelings of personal inadequacy in the face of uncontrollable disease (DHSSPS, 2000).

Unable to respond to questions

Patients and relatives are also likely to ask many questions in response to hearing bad news; the fears of not being able to answer these questions and the fear of the recipient's responses to the answers to these questions are also factors that cause breaking bad news to be a stressful experience.

A SYSTEMATIC APPROACH TO BREAKING BAD NEWS

As with any procedure, giving bad news requires a coherent strategy in order for it to be accomplished successfully (Back *et al.*, 2005). To this effect, protocols and guidelines have been devised (Baile *et al.*, 2000; Vandekieft, 2001; Brixey, 2004). A plan for determining recipients' values, wishes for participation in decision-making and a strategy for addressing their distress when the bad news is disclosed can increase confidence in the task of disclosing unfavourable medical information (Baile *et al.*, 2000).

The majority of guidelines for breaking bad news follow similar steps:

- Preparation for breaking bad news.
- Gathering information.
- Dissemination of knowledge.
- Empathising and responding.
- Summarising and planning for the future.

Preparation for breaking bad news

The first step in breaking bad news is to ensure that you have correctly identified the person who is the recipient of the news. If the patient or relative is unknown to the practitioner, the practitioner should take steps to ensure he or she has the correct person; this is particularly relevant in the case of unexpected death. An example is:

Nurse: Hello, my name is Charge Nurse John Smith, I am caring for Richard Jones. Please excuse my formality, are you Mrs Bridget Jones, Richard's wife?

Where the pathway to death has been through long-term illness, the patient and/or relatives are probably known to the nurse; if this is not the case two questions should be considered:

- Is this nurse the best person to break bad news?
- Is there another nurse or practitioner who knows this patient/ relative well and who could assist in breaking bad news?

Ensure the environment where the discussion is to take place is quiet, private and free from interruptions, and ensure that any mobile communications systems such as bleeps, pagers and mobile telephones are switched off. If any unforeseen interruptions do occur apologise for these. It should be anticipated that the recipient may be upset; providing tissues may be appropriate. It may be appropriate for recipients to choose where they want to be to receive information. If a private room is not available, curtains may be used to obtain some privacy; other staff in the clinical area should be aware that 'bad news' is being discussed and should prevent interruption/distraction.

For example:

Nurse: Mr Smith, I have the results of your recent tests; do you wish to go somewhere private to discuss these?

The way in which Mr Smith answers this question may indicate some expectation of bad news both verbally and non-verbally. In the example below, Mr Smith appears to except the worst; however, the practitioner reassumes some control over the process and ensures that bad news is broken in an appropriate place:

Nurse: Mr Smith, I have the results of you recent tests; do you wish to go somewhere private to discuss these?
Mr Smith: It's bad news isn't it; do I have cancer?
Nurse: I think, Mr Smith, that we should discuss this in private, let us use this room.

The environment should provide room for the nurse and recipient to sit facing each other and reasonably close so that eye contact can be maintained. Sitting down is the preferred posture when breaking bad news and practitioners who do so are rated more highly on overall impression (Bruera *et al.*, 2007). Standing could imply that you do not have time to spend with the recipient and may induce a feeling of inferiority.

Sometimes when breaking bad news to families, several family members may wish to attend the discussion; this could make the situation difficult as the practitioner will not be able to support all family members and will have difficulty maintaining eye contact with all. Identifying key family members may be difficult, but efforts should be made to speak, in the first instance, to the patient's next of kin. This person may also suggest who he or she would like to be there during the discussion. These individuals can then cascade information. Provision should be made, however, to answer any questions other family members may have.

One practitioner only is required to break news, but another practitioner might accompany the first, to provide additional support for the family. A common practice is a nurse accompanying a doctor, as nursing staff may have an established relationship with that particular patient. This also provides an excellent opportunity for learning, as one practitioner can analyse and constructively criticise the process. It can also provide support for the person breaking bad news.

Gathering information

This is the process of exploring what patients know about their condition, in order to allow the practitioner to assess what is already understood so that the information to be delivered is added to and is in congruence with that information. Open-ended questioning is classically used in this stage of discussion; it allows the practitioner to assess at what level to deliver information. For example the recipient may demonstrate some medical background or a comprehensive understanding of the illness. This is frequently seen with transplant patients and those with chronic disease processes such as renal failure.

It may be that the recipient has already been seen by another practitioner, and the pathway to breaking bad news has been prepared, for example a patient who has had a catastrophic head injury whose relatives have met with another practitioner to inform them about pending brain stem death testing.

The process of gathering information also allows the practitioner to clarify any confusion or misconceptions about a condition or events.

Some examples of open-ended questions used at this stage are given below.

Example 1

Nurse: Mrs Smith, what do you understand about your husband's illness?

Mrs Smith: Well, he said he had this lump in his throat that he went to the doctors about.

Nurse: Did he tell you what his doctor said?

Example 2

Nurse: Mr Wood, may I ask what you have been told already about your wife's accident?

The process of gathering information provides an opportunity to obtain consent to breaking bad news and to explore how much the recipient wants to know. Evidence indicates that patients increasingly want additional information regarding their diagnosis, their chances of cure, the side-effects of therapy and a realistic estimate of how long they have to live (Sutherland *et al.*, 1989; Meredith *et al.*, 1996).

However, this thirst for information is not universal, especially as the disease progresses and patients want to focus on 'What do we do next?' (Back *et al.*, 2005). If patients do not want to know details, offers should be made to answer any questions the patient may have in the future (Baile *et al.*, 2000).

Dissemination of knowledge

Knowledge should be disseminated to patients and relatives in a language that is understood by them, which means avoiding medical terminology (Back *et al.*, 2005). Certain phrases/expressions should be avoided as these could lead to confusion, for example if the information that is to be delivered to loved ones is that their relative has died, expression such as 'passed on' or 'slipped away' may be misinterpreted. It may be helpful to give the recipient some advance warning that they are about to receive bad news as this can allow them to prepare psychologically (Back *et al.*, 2005; Buckman, 2005).

Nurse: Mrs Williams, I am afraid I have some rather bad news for you.

The information should be delivered in small portions, at the recipient's pace, allowing the individual time to 'digest' and understand that information. This process may require reiteration and clarification, to check the individual's understanding during the discussion. The information should be delivered honestly but avoiding bluntness, as this is likely to leave the recipient isolated and angry, with a tendency to blame the messenger (DHSSPS, 2000). For example:

Nurse: I am afraid, Mr Able, that you have very bad cancer and unless you get treatment you are going to die.

This may be better presented as:

Nurse: Mr Able, I am sorry to say that the cancer that you have is very aggressive and particularly difficult to treat.
Mr Able: Am I going to die?
Nurse: I am afraid that very few people survive this sort of cancer and if I am honest I think that you will die as a result of it.
Mr Able: Is there any chance of me beating it?
Nurse: I would like to discuss with you some treatment that gives you a small hope, but I cannot guarantee that this will get rid of the cancer.

After breaking the main component of the bad news, stay quiet for few moments. Allow the recipient time to absorb the information and respond (Back *et al.*, 2005); during this time observe their actions/responses. Even if bad news is expected, there will be an element of shock when it is put into words. Recipients need time before they are ready to proceed.

Empathising and responding

Empathy can be described as the power of understanding or imaginatively entering another person's feelings (*Collins English Dictionary*, 1998). Showing empathy, exploring the recipient's understanding and acceptance of what he or she has just learned and validating that person's feelings can provide much-needed support (Buckman, 2005).

An empathetic approach to responding to recipients of bad news is emotionally difficult. The ability to empathise is influenced by personal experiences such as having dealt with loss, and experiences of bereavement. Yet having had such experiences does not necessarily make a person provide empathy more effectively.

It is impossible to understand an individual's relationships with another and thus impossible to imaginatively enter that person's feelings. However, there are certain approaches that allow practitioners to empathise more effectively, and these are based on exploring a person's feelings with them. Buckman (2005) suggests three key steps in providing empathy:

- *Step 1:* Listen for and identify the emotions. This step uses verbal and non-verbal communication, in particular observation of body language, to ascertain what emotion the recipient is experiencing.
- *Step 2:* Identify the cause or source of the emotion, which is most likely to be the bad news that the recipient has just heard. However, there may be underlying emotions such as guilt and blame.
- *Step 3:* Show the recipient that you have made the connection between the above two steps–that you have identified the emotion and its origin.

Utilising this approach can reduce patients' or relatives' isolation, expresses solidarity and validates their feelings or thoughts as normal and to be expected (Ptacek & Eberhardt, 1996).

Some examples of exploring patients' or relatives' feelings are:

Nurse: I can see you are very angry about what I have told you …

or

Nurse: You are obviously very shocked by this information. …

Encourage and allow recipients time to express their emotions and let them know you are trying to understand and acknowledge their emotions. Deliberate periods of silence can allow recipients to process bad news and vent their emotions (Mueller, 2002).

Summarising and planning for the future

This is the process where the summary of the information is given, to ensure that all points are understood and the pathway for future management is discussed. This may be further testing or discussion of treatment options or discussions about end-of-life care. Patients who have a clear plan for the future are less likely to feel anxious and uncertain (Baile *et al.*, 2000) Written materials (e.g. handwritten notes or prepared materials listing the diagnosis and treatment options) may be helpful in some circumstances (Mueller, 2002).

The opportunity for a further discussion should be offered to the recipient. The recipient should also be advised who to approach, in the first instance, with any questions that might arise. Many recipients of bad news need time to digest the information and time to consider options regarding their future, thus an opportunity to discuss matters further after this time will usually be required.

In discussing management plans, the expression 'I am afraid there is little else that can be done' should be avoided as this is inconsistent with the fact that patients often have other important therapeutic goals such as effective pain control, symptom relief and identifying spiritual needs.

RESPONSES TO GRIEF AND RECEIVING BAD NEWS

Generally, grief is associated with the death of a loved one. However, the term may be associated with response to receiving any bad news that has significant influences on health (and its deterioration) and how this event changes that individual's life.

As previously stated, what individuals perceive as bad news will be different and influenced by many factors. Common factors perceived as bad news include an alteration to body image, a reliance on long-term medical/nursing care such as haemodialysis and diagnosis of a life-limiting disease such as cancer or chronic organ system failure. Thus, in exploring responses to grief, it must be considered that the trigger for these responses may be different in each individual.

A large volume of work looking at patients' attitudes and responses towards death and dying or dealing with catastrophic news is influenced by the work of Elisabeth Kübler-Ross (1969), who suggested that patients journey through stages of grief (although not necessarily sequentially). Whilst the model has been criticised as being too rigid and subject to misinterpretation (Germain, 1980); it does suggest the following five common responses to grief that can be observed in a large proportion of patients who receive bad news:

- *Denial,* 'It can't be happening'; the initial stage of shock and numbness, a conscious or unconscious refusal to accept facts.
- *Anger,* 'Why me?'; anger may be internalised or externalised against the clinician, family or the individual's God.
- *Bargaining:* 'Just let me live to see my grandchild born'.
- *Depression:* the initial stages of acceptance.
- *Acceptance:* a stage where there may be some emotional detachment and objectivity.

Kübler-Ross (1969) suggests that patients can move back and forth through stages, become fixated on one stage or can miss stages out completely; this movement is highly individualised and fluidic. The individual responses in each stage can manifest themselves in many different ways. Factors that influence this manifestation can include religion, faith, age, culture, social networks, finances and personal beliefs. Each of the five stages of grief will now be discussed in detail.

Denial
Denial is a conscious or subconscious refusal to accept facts, information and the reality of the situation. It is characteristically an initial response to grief. This may be expressed as: 'It can't be happening' or 'There must have been some mistake'. Denial is usually a temporary defence and is usually replaced by a partial acceptance, although some individuals may still use this as a coping strategy throughout their illness (Kübler-Ross, 1969). Relatives are often happy for a patient to be in denial, as this puts off the day when painful issues have to be faced. They may argue that there is 'time enough' to face reality when the patient becomes weaker (Faulkner, 1998).

Dealing with ongoing denial is particularly difficult; nurses have a responsibility not to lie to patients and would not be acting in their best interests by encouraging denial. However, it is a coping strategy for those patients. Patients should be assisted to accept the 'event' as a mechanism of open questioning to allow patients to re-explore their own feelings. An example of this is given below.

Mr Johns is approaching the end of his life through incurable cancer and he is possibly attempting to get the nurse to collude with his denial:

Mr Johns: Nurse, I have this holiday brochure for a trip next year, what do you think about Poland?

Nurse: Poland looks fantastic Mr Johns, do you think you will be well enough to go next year?

Mr Johns: I should think so once I am over this.

Nurse: When Dr Martin spoke with you and your family last week, he mentioned that he thought the tumour was spreading, do you recall this?

Mr Johns: Yes he did say something about it.

Nurse: Dr Martin said that he did not think he could cure the cancer, I am just wondering how you think your health will be early next year.

Anger

Anger, a very common response to bad news and grief, is often linked to feelings of guilt and blame. Anger can manifest in different ways. People dealing with emotional upset can be angry with themselves and/or with others, especially those close to them.

Some individuals express anger at their religion or belief values. In this case, the nurse may wish to involve a chaplain/spiritual leader in discussions with the patient (this should only be done with the patient's consent).

Anger may be aimed at healthcare professionals, particularly when the cause of illness is uncertain or unknown. Difficult questions may be raised such as 'Why was this not diagnosed earlier?', or 'Why did my own doctor not pick this up?' Attempts should be made to rationalise the process leading up to diagnosis/bad news, which might involve specialist/senior staff.

In dealing with anger, the nurse should establish the cause, whether it is justified and where it is focused. The individual can then be encouraged to locate the true cause of anger, resulting in a healthy discharge of feelings rather than a continuation of unfocused anger (Faulkner, 1998). Nurses should accept a cause of anger if appropriate, but must be careful not to direct blame.

Bargaining

The bargaining stage tends to occur only for short periods of time as it rarely provides a relief from grief and may be directed in a spiritual way: 'If God has decided to take me away and he did not respond to my angry pleas, perhaps he will be more favourable if I ask politely' or 'If I stop smoking now perhaps the cancer will go away'. Bargaining, in reality, is a process of trying to postpone what in many cases is inevitable.

Depression

This stage characteristically occurs when denial and anger have given way to a sense of great loss (Kübler-Ross, 1969); it can be manifested further by a deterioration in physical health/ability/ independence. This process may be an indication that a patient has begun to accept the reality of the situation.

Acceptance

Acceptance is the stage where a patient is neither depressed nor angry about his or her fate. People approaching the end of life can enter this stage a long time before their loved ones, a fact that the latter can find emotionally distressing.

Other responses to grief

Other responses to grief include:

- Low or sad mood.
- Insomnia.
- Decreased appetite.
- Irritability.
- Guilt or self-criticism.

It is important to remember that many patients and their families experience stages of grief such as those suggested by Kübler-Ross, but will do so individually. For example, relatives of a patient who is in acceptance of his condition may still be in denial; this situation can create difficulties in communication.

How the pathway to death alters responses to grief

The stages described above may be experienced by many individuals as they deal with grief, but time may not allow for this in patients where death is a result of a catastrophic event such as a road accident or fatal myocardial infarction. Many individuals who meet death this way are, or become, unconscious during emergency care, thus responding to grief, as outlined above, does not occur. However, relatives of these individuals respond to grief, perhaps with a greater emphasis on anger and denial, as the event is thrust on them with no warning and no psychological adaptation time, or time to spend with the dying person.

Consideration must also be given to those with communication difficulties who are impeded in their ability to express themselves, for example awake patients on ventilatory support.

BREAKING BAD NEWS FOLLOWING AN UNEXPECTED DEATH

The principles of breaking bad news to relatives following the unexpected death of a loved one are very similar to those described above. However, there are two important points to note:

- When breaking bad news following an unsuccessful resuscitation attempt: ensure a presentable appearance, e.g. check the clothing for blood, wash hands, etc (Resuscitation Council UK, 2006).
- It is particularly important to be perfectly frank very early on in the conversation therefore use an unambiguous term, e.g. dead, died or death, and repeat it at least once more to reinforce it. Do not 'beat around the bush'; relatives will want to know immediately whether their loved one is alive or dead (Resuscitation Council UK, 2006). Avoid using ambiguous language, e.g. 'We have lost him' or 'He has gone to a better place'; this vague terminology can be misinterpreted.

The relatives' response to the bad news could include:

- Acute emotional distress/shock.
- Anger.
- Disbelief.
- Guilt.
- Catatony.

(Resuscitation Council UK, 2006)

CONCLUSION

This chapter has provided an overview to the principles of breaking bad news. The objectives of breaking bad news have been listed and effective communication skills outlined. Barriers to breaking bad news effectively have been explored and a systematic approach to breaking bad news has been described. The responses to grief and receiving bad news have been discussed. Guidelines for breaking bad news following an unexpected death have been outlined.

REFERENCES

Back AL, Arnold RM, Baile WF, Tulsky JA, Fryer-Edwards K (2005) Approaching difficult communication tasks in oncology, *Cancer J Clin* **55**: 164–177.

Baile WF, Buckman R, Lenzi R, Glober G, Beale EA, Kudelka AP (2000) SPIKES – A six-step protocol for delivering bad news: Application to the patient with cancer. *Oncologist* **5**: 302–311.

Brixey L (2004) The difficult task of delivering bad news. *Dermatol Nurs.* **16**(4): 347–358.

Bruera E, Palmer JL, Pace E, *et al.* (2007) A randomized, controlled trial of physician postures when breaking bad news to cancer patients. *Palliat Med* **21**: 501–505.

Buckman R (1984) Breaking bad news: Why is it still so difficult? *BMJ* **288**(6430): 1597–1599.

Buckman RA (2005) Breaking bad news: The S-P-I-K-E-S strategy. *Community Oncol* **2**(2): 138–142.

Collins English Dictionary Millennium Edition (1998) Harper Collins Publishers, Glasgow.

Department of Health, Social Services & Public Safety (DHSSPS) (2000) *Breaking Bad News. Regional Guidelines*, DHSSPS Belfast.

Faulkner A (1998) ABC of palliative care: Communication with patients, families, and other professionals. *BMJ* **316**: 130–132.

Germain CP (1980) Nursing the dying: implications of Kübler-Ross' staging theory. *Ann Am Acad Pol Soc Sci* **447**: 46.

Hall A (2005) Breaking bad news. *J Community Nurs* **19**(9): 30–31.

Holland JC (1989) Now we tell – But how well. *J Clin Oncol* **7**: 557–559.

Kübler-Ross E (1969) *On death and dying.* Macmillan, New York.

Meredith C, Symond P, Webster L, *et al.* (1996) Information needs of cancer patients in West Scotland: Cross sectional survey of patients' views. *BMJ* **313**: 724–726.

Mueller PS (2002) Breaking bad news to patients: The 'SPIKES' approach can make this difficult task easier. *Postgrad Med* **112**(3): 15–18.

Ptacek JT, Eberhardt TL (1996) Breaking bad news: A review of the literature. *J Am Med Assoc* **276**(6): 496–502.

Resuscitation Council UK (2006) *Advanced Life Support*, 5th edn. Resuscitation Council UK, London.

Sutherland HJ, Llewellyn-Thomas HA, Lockwood GA, Tritchler DL, Till JE (1989) Cancer patients: Their desire for information and participation in treatment decisions. *J R Soc Med* **82**: 260–263.

Vandekieft GK (2001) Breaking bad news. *Am Fam Physician* **64**(12): 1975–1978.

9 | Last Offices

Dan Higgins

INTRODUCTION

The term 'last offices' relates to the care of a body after death, with specific regard to the procedures involved in preparing for transfer to a chapel of rest, mortuary or undertakers. It is a process that demonstrates respect for the dead and is focused on fulfilling religious and cultural beliefs as well as health and safety and legal requirements (Dougherty & Lister, 2004). Terms associated with last offices include 'laying out' and 'preparing the body'.

Administering last offices often has symbolic significance for nurses and can be a fulfilling experience as it is the final demonstration of respectful, sensitive care given to a patient (Nearney, 1998a).

The aim of this chapter is to understand how to perform last offices.

LEARNING OUTCOMES

At the end of this chapter, the reader will be able to:

❏ List the objectives of performing last offices.
❏ Discuss the importance of respecting the patient's dignity.
❏ Outline infection control issues.
❏ Discuss the legal issues.
❏ Discuss the religious, cultural and spiritual considerations.
❏ Outline the procedure for the performance of last offices.

OBJECTIVES OF PERFORMING LAST OFFICES

The objectives of last offices are to:

• Ensure that the body is treated with the utmost dignity and respect.

- Prevent the spread of infection from the deceased to staff, other patients and those involved in afterlife care, such as mortuary staff.
- Prepare the body to look as 'peaceful as possible'.
- Comply with legal guidelines for afterlife care.
- Ensure that any spiritual, religious and cultural preferences expressed by the patient, in life or by his or her loved ones are adhered to.
- Facilitate safe transfer to destination, generally the mortuary/ chapel of rest or undertakers.

THE IMPORTANCE OF RESPECTING THE PATIENT'S DIGNITY

The Nursing and Midwifery Council (NMC) code of professional conduct (NMC, 2002) states:

> 'You are personally accountable for ensuring that you promote and protect the interests and dignity of patients and clients, irrespective of gender, age, race, ability, sexuality, economic status, lifestyle, culture and religious or political beliefs.'

The Code (NMC, 2008) reiterates the importance of treating patients as individuals and respecting their dignity. This should be upheld following death; patients (and their loved ones) must be treated with the respect and dignity they were provided with prior to death. This requires the last offices to be performed as if attending to the needs of live patients.

Some nurses 'talk to the patient' during last offices, which some may find uncomfortable, and some perform the procedure in silence. If relatives are present or involved in the procedure, their feelings on such matters should be sought. Any wishes or preferences that the patient expressed prior to death should be honoured, for example a patient requesting that his or her wedding ring is not removed after death. Preferences expressed by the patient's loved ones should also be respected, as events may influence their grieving processes.

In line with treating the patient with respect and dignity, all efforts should be made to ensure the patient looks 'peaceful'. Unless contraindicated or against the relatives' wishes, attempts should be made to close the patient's eyes and mouth. Any evidence of blood/body fluids marking the body, in particular on the face, should be removed. Vascular lines, catheters and tubes should be removed unless legal requirements dictate otherwise. Many relatives wish to view the body in the chapel of rest following transfer from the place of death, and creating a peaceful impression may aid the grieving process.

There are certain circumstances where death has occurred and legal requirements, such as referral to a coroner and/or postmortem examination, will be required. This influences last offices practice, most notably preventing the removal of invasive lines and tubes. Circumstances where this may occur will be explored later in this text.

INFECTION CONTROL ISSUES

The deceased poses no greater threat of an infection risk than when alive, but natural leakage of body fluids could occur and the risk of transfer of pathogens is high. In the majority of infective cases, the universal precautions (see Box 9.1) that were in place prior to death will be sufficient to prevent cross-infection post death. However, certain modifications to the last offices procedure may be required including:

Box 9.1 Universal infection control procedures when performing last offices

- Optimum hand hygiene
- Use of personal protective equipment, such as gloves/aprons
- Safe handling and disposal of sharps
- Safe handling and disposal of clinical waste as per organisational policy
- Safe management of blood and bodily fluids, for example spillages
- Decontamination of any equipment
- Maintaining a clean clinical environment
- Good communication with other healthcare workers, patients and visitors

Adapted from Royal College of
Nursing (RCN) (2005)

- Eye and face protection if there is a risk of splashing.
- The use of a body bag where gross leakage of blood and body fluids is suspected.
- The use of 'danger of infection' labels, although the rationale for this must be discussed with relatives otherwise offence may be caused.
- The use of body bags for certain infectious diseases (see Box 9.2).
- Communication with senior mortuary staff prior to transfer of the body regarding infective status.

The UK today is a multicultural and multi-faith society, this is a great challenge to nurses, who need to be aware of the different religious and cultural rituals that may accompany the death of a patient (Dougherty & Lister, 2004). Whilst these rituals/ approaches are a very important component of respectful and dignified afterlife care, applying such rituals as a blanket policy may be against patients' wishes/best interests. Discussion of performing last offices for individuals from different faiths and cultures is explored later in this text, but meeting the patient's and his or her family's needs effectively after death can only be

---

Box 9.2 Infectious disease processes requiring extra infection control procedures in addition to universal precautions

- Human immundeficiency virus (HIV)
- Acquired immune deficiency syndrome (AIDS)
- Hepatitis B virus (Hep B)
- Hepatitis C virus (Hep C)
- Creutzfeldt–Jakob disease and other transmissible spongiform encephalopathies
- Tuberculosis
- Meningococcal septicaemia
- Invasive group A Streptococcal infection
- Viral haemorrhagic fevers

In all cases of infectious disease advice from infection control staff should be sought.

---

achieved through excellent communication with that patient, in life, and/or the family.

Once last offices have been performed, the body will require transfer to the mortuary. This process should involve excellent communication between portering staff, mortuary staff and those responsible for last offices in order for the patient to be transferred safely and in consideration of other patients. Clear documentation is of paramount importance at this stage, as care is effectively being handed over.

LEGAL ISSUES

The nurse's responsibility to the deceased patient remains until the body leaves his or her clinical environment for the mortuary. This requires that communication with the family and the last offices procedure are documented in full to provide a record of care. The nurse also has a responsibility for the health and safety of colleagues in the clinical area. This requires minimising the risk of cross-infection, as discussed earlier, and recognising any distress caused to others by that patient's death.

Death must be verified prior to the commencement of last offices. This process has traditionally been undertaken by a medical practitioner, but nurses who have undertaken the required training may verify death in certain cases. The verification process is legal confirmation that the patient has died and should be documented accordingly. Last offices can then be performed.

Following verification of death, a medical certificate stipulating the cause of death should be completed by a doctor who has attended the deceased during his or her last illness. The medical certificate of cause of death is delivered by the 'informant' (usually the next of kin) to the Registrar of Births and Deaths, who issues the death certificate. Under certain situations, the registrar has a statutory obligation to refer the death to the coroner. A coroner is an independent judicial officer who is responsible for investigating violent, unnatural deaths or sudden deaths of unknown cause and deaths in custody that are reported to him/her.

The registrar has a duty to refer deaths to the coroner if:

- The deceased had not been seen by the doctor within 14 days of the death.
- The certifying doctor had not seen the body after death.
- The cause of death is unknown.
- Death was violent or unnatural or suspicious.
- Death may be due to an accident (whenever it occurred).
- Death may be due to self-neglect or neglect by others.
- Death may be due to an industrial disease or related to the deceased's employment.
- Death may be due to an abortion.
- Death occurred during an operation or before recovery from the effects of an anaesthetic.
- Death may be a suicide.
- Death occurred during or shortly after detention in police or prison custody.

(Adapted from Department of Health (DH), 2007)

Certain factors, such as the placement of vascular access lines, tubes and monitoring devices, may have contributed to the death of a patient; as such, they must be left *in situ* pending referral to the coroner. Medical staff should always be consulted about removing lines and their response documented.

Access devices and lines if left *in situ* may cause some distress to relatives if they wish to view the body following last offices. Gauze and adhesive tape may be used as a cover; large bore tubes such as intercostal drains can be cut and spigoted. An explanation should be given to any relatives of the rationale behind this practice.

In certain environments, for example intensive care units, devices such as tracheal tubes may be removed prior to last offices so that family members can spend time with their relative without a plethora of medical equipment. This should only occur with the consent of senior medical staff.

CULTURAL, RELIGIOUS AND SPIRITUAL CONSIDERATIONS

Practices relating to last offices vary depending on the patient's cultural background and religious practices (Nearney, 1998b). Whilst the discussion below outlines some of the major cultural/

religious preferences regarding last offices, it would be insensitive to apply these as a blanket policy for a particular cultural group because some individuals are not whole-hearted in acceptance of the ways of that individual's religious or cultural group (Neuberger, 1999).

The given religion of a patient may occasionally be offered to indicate an association with particular cultural and national roots, rather than to indicate a significant degree of adherence to the tenets of a particular faith (Dougherty & Lister, 2004). Nursing care can be improved, however, with knowledge about the traditions and beliefs of patients in certain cultural and religious groups (Neuberger, 2004). Optimum care in last offices can only be achieved when pre-existing knowledge is complemented by discussion with the patients, in life, or their family after death, as to what their specific needs are.

Specific issues relating to performing last offices in patients with varying religions will now be discussed.

Christians, including Roman Catholics

There are no specific modifications to last offices practice for deceased patients of the Christian faith, although the family should be consulted as certain groups may have specific requirements. Christian families do not tend to become directly involved in the last offices procedure but, as with all groups, relatives should be given the opportunity to participate if requested (Cooke, 2000). After consultation with relatives, it may be necessary to contact the appropriate hospital chaplain. Sometimes it may be necessary to contact the patient's own priest or vicar. Small items such as a crucifix, holy picture or rosary beads may be placed near the patient or in the patient's hands (Green, 1993).

The sacrament of anointing of the sick (sometimes referred to as last rites) has as its purpose the conferral of a special grace on the Christian experiencing the difficulties inherent in the condition of grave illness or old age; only priests (presbyters and bishops) can administer the sacrament of the anointing of the sick, using oil blessed by the bishop, or if necessary by the celebrating presbyter himself (The Vatican, 2008).

Anointing of the sick is usually undertaken in those who are critically ill or very near to death, although sometimes it is undertaken immediately following death. It consists of the anointing of the forehead and hands of the sick person (in the Roman rite) or of other parts of the body (in the Eastern rite), the anointing being accompanied by the liturgical prayer of the celebrant asking for the special grace of this sacrament (the Vatican, 2008).

Islam (Muslim)

When a Muslim is making his or her final gasps, the relatives give holy water (zam zam) and verses from the Quraan are read (Gatrad, 1994). After death, a Muslim patient should not be touched by non-Muslim hands; healthcare workers, following consultation with the family, should wear disposable gloves (Green, 1991).

In death, it is preferred that the face is facing Mecca (the religious centre for Muslims and place of religious pilgrimage); in the UK, Mecca is in the east. In hospitals, it is considered acceptable if the head is turned to the right (so the body can be buried with the face towards Mecca) (Green, 1991). The arms and legs should be straightened and the mouth and eyes closed. A bandage tied around the chin is required to hold the mouth closed. All clothes should be removed by a person of the same sex and the body covered with a sheet (Gatrad, 1994).

The body should not be washed as this is undertaken by respected Muslim elders experienced in Muslim burial. This generally occurs in the home or mosque, although transfer from the clinical environment to the mortuary is acceptable. If the body is to be washed in the healthcare setting by Muslim elders, advice may be given about health and safety/infection issues.

Burial (never cremation) should take place as soon as possible, preferably within 24 h; any delays (such as coroner's referral) can cause distress to the family. However, the law takes precedence, although this may require sensitive communication with the relatives. If coroner's referral is required, the office should be informed to facilitate a speedy release of the death certificate. This may also facilitate release of the body as certain groups may wish to transport the body to the country of origin for burial.

Hinduism

The family should be consulted regarding preferences prior to the commencement of last offices as some may object to the body being touched by 'non-Hindu hands' and many relatives may wish to take the body home for ritual washing. If last offices are to be performed in an inpatient setting many Hindus express a preference that passages from the Bhagavad Gita (the Hindu holy text) are read aloud; this may be performed by a Hindu priest/relative or a member of staff (Green, 1991). Relatives may wish to be present during last offices.

Any special threads or jewellery should be left *in situ*; this should be included on the 'notification of death' documents to advise mortuary staff. If relatives are unavailable, the patient's limbs should be straightened and the eyes closed (wearing disposable gloves). The body should not be washed, but wrapped in a plain sheet. Requests may be made to dress the body in normal clothes and for holy water to be added to the water being used to wash the body.

Adult Hindus are generally cremated and there is a preference for this process to occur as quickly as possible (preferably within 24h). Excellent communication will be required should delays occur.

Sikhism

Generally, Sikhs are happy for non-Sikhs to perform last offices, but relatives, particularly the eldest son, may wish to be involved or perform the procedure themselves (Green, 1991). Relatives or a priest may want to sit by the patient and read from the Holy Guru Granth Sahib (holy book).

Central to 'confirmed' Sikh belief are the five Ks, which are:

- *Kesh:* uncut hair (including the beard) and covering the hair at all times, usually with a turban; hair is considered the most sacred part of the body and should be treated with respect.
- *Kanga:* a semi-circular comb that fixes hair.
- *Kara:* a steel bracelet worn on the right wrist (the circular shape reminds the wearer of the unity of God and the community of Sikhs); a constant and visible reminder to Sikhs that all their actions should be righteous.

- *Kaccha:* a particular type of undergarment worn by both men and women; devout Sikhs wear the Kaccha day and night, never removing it.
- *Kirpan:* a dagger symbolising the Sikhs' readiness to fight in self-defence or to protect the oppressed; in the UK most Sikhs only wear a small symbolic kirpan.

These five Ks should be left intact during last offices and not removed unless specifically requested. During the procedure, the arms and legs should be straightened and the mouth and eyes closed, and the body should be covered in a plain white sheet or a shroud.

Sikh funerals should usually take place within 24 h or as soon as possible. Thus the coroner's office should be informed, if referral is to be made, to hasten proceedings as much as possible. Sensitive communication will be required should delays occur.

Judaism

If death occurs during the Sabbath (commencing before nightfall on a Friday and ending on the Saturday evening (Green, 1991), the body should not be touched until the Sabbath has ended; however, this is impractical in most healthcare settings and as such last offices are generally performed.

The eyes are usually closed following death; a member of family may wish to perform this task. The body should not be washed but covered and left untouched. It is generally accepted that healthcare staff are permitted to perform any procedure for preserving dignity and honour, although this must be done wearing gloves and by touching the body as little as possible. These procedures may include attending to hygiene needs for soiling, and the removal of lines and access devices, unless contraindicated (Dougherty & Lister, 2004). Last offices are generally performed by a Jewish undertaker or the synagogue personnel prior to burial.

Burial should usually take place as soon as possible (preferably within 24 h), although this may be delayed for the Sabbath, thus the coroner's office should be informed, if referral is to be made, to hasten proceedings as much as possible. Sensitive communication will be required should delays occur. Cremation is not permitted in the Jewish faith.

Buddhism
There are no specific modifications to last offices practice for Buddhists, although the family should be consulted as certain groups may have specific requirements. It is of paramount importance that when a Buddhist dies, the Buddhist minister, monk or sister is contacted as soon as possible. In the absence of family, and if practical, it may be wise to not commence last offices until this time. The body should not be moved until a Buddhist priest has prayed over the body.

Baha'i faith
There are no specific modifications to last offices practice for deceased patients of Baha'i faith, although the family should be consulted as certain groups may have specific requirements; this may include a ring placed on the finger of the body, which should not be removed (Dougherty & Lister, 2004).

Baha'is are always buried, never cremated (Green, 1991) and the place of internment should be at a place within 1 h's journey from the place of death.

Christian Scientists
There are no specific modifications to last offices practice for deceased patients of the Christian Scientists faith, although the family should be consulted as certain groups may have specific requirements.

Jehovah's Witnesses
There are no specific modifications to last offices practice for deceased patients of the Jehovah's Witness faith, although the family should be consulted as certain groups may have specific requirements.

Church of Jesus Christ of the Latter Day Saints (Mormons)
There are no specific modifications to last offices practice for deceased patients of the Church of Jesus Christ of the Latter Day Saints, although the family should be consulted as certain groups

may have specific requirements, including dressing the body in a sacred garment following the procedure.

Zoroastrianism

There are no specific modifications to last offices practice for deceased patients of the Zoroastrianism faith, although the family should be consulted as certain groups may have specific requirements. The family may request that one or two sacred garments are worn next to the skin underneath the shroud and the head be covered with a cap or scarf (Green, 1993).

The funeral should usually take place as soon as possible (preferably within 24 h), thus the coroner's office should be informed, if referral is to be made, to hasten proceedings as much as possible. Again, sensitive communication will be required should delays occur.

Rastafarianism

There are no specific modifications to last offices practice for deceased patients of the Rastafarian faith, although the family should be consulted as certain groups may have specific requirements.

PROCEDURE FOR THE PERFORMANCE OF LAST OFFICES

The following procedure for the performance of last offices is intended as a guide only and should be influenced by the patient's preferences expressed in life and those of the family/significant others, together with local policy. In some situations, relatives may wish to be involved in some aspects of performing last offices, for example helping to wash the body. A standard checklist can help ensure that last offices are undertaken correctly (Figure 9.1).

A suggested procedure for the performance of last offices is as follows:

- Ensure verification of death has been undertaken and documented appropriately. This is to comply with legal requirements and prevent unnecessary coroner's referral.
- Ascertain if the deceased is to be referred to the coroner (this influences decisions regarding removal of lines/devices).

WALSALL HOSPITALS NHS TRUST

Checklist Following Death of a Patient

PATIENT NAME:.. DATE:................................

UNIT NUMBER:..

Labelling of body

Wristband - check information	**Yes/No**
Attach ticket to ankle	**Yes/No**
Attach ticket to shroud	**Yes/No**
Check valuables on body and record on ticket	**Yes/No**
Attach white label in plastic envelope to sheet or body bag/liner	**Yes/No**

Infection control

Leaking wounds / IV sites covered with occlusive dressing	**Yes/No**
If infectious (ie HIV, Hep B) Use body bag and label 'Danger of infection'	**Yes/No**
If infected with MRSA, or similar, or leaking, wrap in body liner (plastic sheet)	**Yes/No**

Property

Clothing and valuables recorded in property book	**Yes/No**

Information

Information booklet to relatives	**Yes/No**
Advice given to relatives to contact General office	**Yes/No**
Inform mortuary re: Use of body bag / liner	**Yes/No**

Signature.. Designation..

(Please file in patient's medical records)

Striving for Excellence in Healthcare

KS/BS/CHECKLIST
September 2001

WZZ 08602

Fig 9.1 Checklist following death of a patient. Reproduced by kind permission of Walsall Hospitals NHS Trust

- Ascertain the need for a body bag and the requirements for any added infection control procedures to comply with organisational health and safety and infection control policies.
- Discuss with the family any specific preferences for last offices.
- Assemble equipment.
- Screen off the bed area – in respect for the deceased and prevent distress to other patients.
- Remove tubes, lines and access devices, as agreed with senior medical staff.
- If they need to remain *in situ*, to improve the relatives' experience of viewing the body post procedure, cut and spigot off any large bore tubes and cover with gauze and adhesive dressing.
- If the patient is not catheterised, apply gentle pressure over the supra-pubic region to facilitate bladder emptying (Cooke, 2000).
- Unless specified otherwise, remove any jewellery etc., witnessed by another member of staff. Ensure all jewellery removed or left on the body is clearly documented.
- Provide full body wash, paying attention to facial shave, hair care, oral care and nail care (Note: When moving/rolling the body, sometimes groaning sounds can be heard as air is expelled out of the lungs).
- Close the eyes (use a small amount of clinical tape on the eyelids if required).
- Place dentures in the mouth if possible. If unable to do this, place them in a pot, label it and send it to the mortuary with the body.
- Dress the body in clothes/gown/shroud as required and as directed by family/previous expressed wishes.
- Attach identification labels (Figure 9.2), as per local policy.
- Place an incontinence sheet underneath the buttocks to contain any faecal/urine soiling.
- If a body bag is not required, enclose the body in a sheet, securing with adhesive tape.
- If a body bag is required, place the body in the bag according to the manufacturer's instructions (a sheet is not ideally used with a body bag as a 'wick' is created).

WALSALL HOSPITALS NHS TRUST

UNIT No. ....

SURNAME ....

FIRST NAME(S)...

ADDRESS ....

....

CONSULTANT ....WARD ....

DATE OF DEATH ....AGE ....
ASMH 18   P.T.O.

VALUABLES ON BODY: YES ☐   NO ☐

**PLEASE LIST VALUABLES ON
NOTIFICATION OF DEATH CARD.**

SIGNATURE OF NURSE IN CHARGE................................

Fig 9.2 Identification labels. Reproduced by kind permission of Walsall Hospitals NHS Trust

- Complete documentation (notification of death) (Figure 9.3) as per organisational policy.
- Document any property of the deceased. Document the last offices procedure and any previous discussion with relatives in the patient's notes.
- Ensure any jewellery/items left on the patient are documented on the notification of death form.
- Dispose of clinical waste following local policy.
- Arrange for transfer of the body, communicating any specific requirements to portering/mortuary staff (it is standard practice to transport the body off the ward/clinical area discreetly).
- If the body is to be transferred to an area other than the mortuary (home/undertakers), ensure that all administrative processes have been completed (involve site co-ordinator/senior nursing management staff).
- Take property, patient records, etc. to general office/bereavement office as per local policy to facilitate administrative processes.

....HOSPITAL, WALSALL

NOTIFICATION OF DEATH

SURNAME		UNIT NUMBER	
FIRST NAME(S)		DATE OF BIRTH	
ADDRESS		CONSULTANT	
		HOSPITAL	
G.P.		WARD	OPD

Date of Death...**Time**.................................

Religion..

**Name and Address of
Next of Kin**..

....

....

Telephone No:...

Present at time of death YES/NO

If already notified   YES/NO

Signed..

Fig 9.3 Notification of death. Reproduced by kind permission of Walsall Hospitals NHS Trust

Performing last offices in the home

Fifty-four per cent of deaths in England and Wales occur in acute hospital beds; 22% of people die at home (Office of National Statistics, 1999). If the patient has died at home through choice (receiving end-of-life care at home), last offices will be performed in that environment. Family members may do this before the undertakers remove the body. There may also be a request that the body is transferred from an organisation into the home environment (for last offices and or viewing), although this is now generally a rare event (Weber *et al.*, 1998). Where appropriate, the ability to perform last offices safely and within legal frameworks should be an essential requirement of primary care services.

Procedure for viewing the body

Viewing the body following last offices may aid the grieving process for some relatives, particularly if they wished to be with the deceased around the time of death but were not. Many relatives wish to see the body to pay their last respects. The facility to do so should be encouraged organisationally, in hospitals (sometimes before transfer of the body from the ward/clinical area), in a chapel of rest or at the undertakers.

In a hospital situation this service may be difficult to arrange, and sensitive communication should be employed as the arrangements to organise this may take a little time. If at all possible relatives should be accompanied by a qualified nurse, preferably the one who cared for the patient/family or somebody with experience in communicating with bereaved relatives, such as a member of the bereavement care team. The responsibility of presenting the body in the chapel of rest usually lies with mortuary staff or out of hours portering staff. The nurse who accompanies the family should check the presentation before the viewing to ensure no factor, such as leakage of body secretions, causes undue distress to the family. The nurse may also forewarn the family of how the body appears, for example 'a little mottled', or 'eyes slightly open', as this may help them prepare psychologically.

The nurse should stay with the family to provide support throughout the viewing and when they have spent enough time, escort the family from the chapel of rest.

CONCLUSION

The aim of this chapter has been to understand how to perform last offices. The objectives of performing last offices have been listed and the importance of respecting the patient's dignity has been discussed. Infection control issues have been highlighted and the legal issues outlined. The religious, cultural and spiritual considerations have been identified and the procedure for the performance of last offices has been described.

The performance of last offices is the delivery of respectful, dignified care following death, in line with individual preference and the preferences of the bereft relatives. Ensuring that the procedure is performed in line with these preferences is a major step in allowing a 'good death' and facilitating the grieving process of relatives/loved ones. The procedure is also bound by legal, health and safety, and organisational guidelines, with which nurses have an obligation to comply. Sensitivity in communication is the primary step to ensure that the final component of care delivered to that patient and subsequent care delivered to the relatives meets these key requirements. In achieving this, a symbolic sense of closure may be achieved by nursing staff, ultimately influencing ongoing practice.

REFERENCES

Cooke H (2000) *When Someone Dies: A Practical Guide to Holistic Care at the End of Life*. Butterworth-Heinemann, Oxford.

Department of Health (DH) (2007) *Consultation on Improving the Process of Death Certification*. Available at www.dh.gov.uk/publications (accessed June 2009).

Dougherty L, Lister S (2004) *The Royal Marsden Hospital Manual of Clinical Nursing Procedures*. 6th edn. Blackwell Publishing, Oxford.

Gatrad A (1994) *The Muslim Patient*. Nursing Times, London

Green J (1991) *Death with Dignity – Meeting the Needs of Patients in a Multi-Cultural Society*. Nursing Times, London.

Green J (1993) *Death with Dignity Volume II – Meeting the Needs of Patients in a Multi-Cultural Society*. Nursing Times, London.

Nearney L (1998a) Practical procedures for nurses. Last Offices, Part 1. *Nursing Times* **94**: 26.

Nearney L (1998b) Practical procedures for nurses. Last Offices, Part 2. *Nursing Times* **94**: 27.

Neuberger J (1999) Cultural issues in palliative care. In: *Oxford Textbook of Palliative Medicine* (eds D Doyle, G Hanks & N MacDonald), pp. 777–801. Oxford University Press, Oxford.

Neuberger J (2004) *Dying Well: A Guide to Enabling a Good Death*. Radcliffe Medical Press, Oxford.

Nursing and Midwifery Council (NMC) (2002) *Code of Professional Conduct*. NMC, London.

Nursing and Midwifery Council (NMC) (2008) *The Code: Standards of Conduct, Performance and Ethics for Nurses and Midwives*. NMC, London.

Office of National Statistics (1999) 1997 *Mortality Statistics, General: England and Wales*. The Stationery Office, London.

Royal College of Nursing (RCN) (2005) *Good Practice in Infection Prevention and Control: Guidance for Nursing Staff*. RCN, London.

Vatican (2008) Catechism of the Catholic Church. Available at www.vatican.va/archive/catechism/p2s2c2a5.htm (accessed 4 December 2008).

Weber M, Ochsmann R, Huber C (1998) Laying out and viewing the body at home – A forgotten tradition? *J Palliat Care* **14**(4): 34–37.

Legal Issues of Death | **10**

Richard Griffith

INTRODUCTION

Some 2000 people die each day in the UK, yet some 1300 of these individuals die without having made a will. People seldom understand the legal framework that regulates what happens to their bodies after death and this can result in their wishes being ignored. In addition, the legal implications of death are rarely discussed by patients, who often find it difficult to talk about their estate and the disposal of their remains.

Difficulty discussing a patient's wishes also extends to decisions at the end of life, particularly where this relates to the continuing or withdrawing of life-sustaining treatment and requests for help to die.

The aim of this chapter is to understand the legal issues of death.

LEARNING OUTCOMES

At the end of the chapter, the reader will be able to:

❏ Discuss a definition of death.
❏ Describe the process of certification and registration of death.
❏ Outline the process for reporting a death to the coroner.
❏ Explain the requirements for verification by nurses of expected death.
❏ Discuss the status of the body after death.
❏ Discuss the issues associated with organ donation.
❏ Discuss the law relating to life-sustaining treatment.
❏ Outlines the issues associated with euthanasia.

DEFINITION OF DEATH

There is no definition of death that is spelt out in statute law (Kennedy & Grubb, 1998). Generally, the Triad of Bichat is used to determine if a person has died (Mason & McCall Smith, 1994).

This defines death as, 'The failure of the body as an integrated system associated with the irreversible loss of circulation, respiration and innervation'. The definition requires a doctor or other health professional to verify that death has occurred by confirming that irreversible loss of circulation, respiration and innervation has taken place.

Advances in medical technology and mechanical ventilation have led to the courts also accepting in evidence that a person is dead when there is death of the brain stem. In *Re A* (1992), a child was admitted to hospital with serious injuries that led the doctors to agree that he was brain stem dead and asked the parents for permission to switch off the life support. A family proceeding court ordered that the parents could not consent to the doctors switching off life support. However, the High Court declared that the child was dead and the doctors would not be acting unlawfully if they disconnected the child from the ventilator.

The administrative system for confirming death relies heavily on the opinion of a doctor to corroborate that a person has died. The general approach of the law is best summed up by Lord Lane in *R v Malcherek & Steel* [1981]. He held that:

> 'Where a medical practitioner adopting methods which are generally accepted comes bona fide and conscientiously to the conclusion that the patient is for practical purposes dead then the courts will accept that the patient is dead.'

> (Lord Lane at 429)

Essentially then, in law a person is dead when a doctor says so. Such a system requires checks and balances in place to prevent wrongdoing. Therefore, there is a duty on the registered medical practitioner attending the patient during his or her last illness or who sees the body after death to issue a medical certificate of cause of death and the death must be registered with the local registrar of births, deaths and marriages (Births and Deaths Registration Act, 1953, section 22).

THE PROCESS OF CERTIFICATION AND REGISTRATION OF DEATH

Before a death can be registered, a properly completed medical certificate of cause of death and a formal notice of death must be issued by the doctor who has provided care during the last illness and who has seen the deceased within 14 days of death or has seen the body after death. The doctor must be confident about the cause of death.

The certificate of cause of death is given to the personal representative or family representative, who must take it to the local registrar of births, deaths and marriages. Where the registrar has the information to complete the entry into the death register and decides that the death does not need reporting to the coroner then he or she will issue:

- A certificate for burial or cremation.
- A certificate of registration of death (required for social security purposes).

Where requested, copies of the entry in the death register, usually called the death certificate, are issued. Two copies of the death certificate are generally required by the person's representative in order to show banks and insurance companies when settling the person's affairs.

If the body is to be buried in England and Wales then no further formalities are required. Where the burial is to be outside of England and Wales then only the coroner can give permission for the body to be moved. This generally requires four days' notice and the coroner will issue a removal notice allowing the movement of the body.

Where there is to be burial at sea, a removal notice and a licence from the Department of Fisheries, Agriculture and Food is required and the District Inspector of Fisheries must be notified (Home Office, 2003).

Cremation certificate

In the case of cremation, the person's representative or family representative must make an application for cremation and the doctor who provided the medical certificate of cause of death completes the cremation form along with a second doctor, not in the same practice as the first who has been qualified for more than five years.

This second doctor is now required to contact the person caring for the deceased to ask if there are any concerns about the medical management of the deceased. The second doctor is only able to complete the cremation form after seeing the body and discussing the death with the first doctor and any person present at the time of death (The Shipman Inquiry, 2004).

This properly completed medical certificate is then generally given to the funeral director, who takes it to the medical referee at the chosen crematorium, who checks the forms and gives the final approval necessary for cremation to occur.

REPORTING A DEATH TO THE CORONER

Occasionally, circumstances occur in which the death must be reported to the coroner. The coroner is a doctor or lawyer responsible for investigating deaths in the following situations:

- The deceased was not attended by a doctor during the last illness or the doctor treating the deceased had not seen the person either after death or within the 14 days before death.
- The death was violent or unnatural or occurred under suspicious circumstances.
- The cause of death is not known or is uncertain.
- The death occurred while the patient was undergoing an operation or did not recover from the anaesthetic.
- The death was caused by an industrial disease.
- The death occurred in prison or in police custody.

(For a more considered discussion of the role of the coroner see Chapter 12).

Under the provisions of the Registration of Births and Death Regulations 1987, the person with a statutory duty to report a death to the coroner is the registrar (see Box 10.1).

It is, however, considered good practice for a doctor to report a death to the coroner directly. It reduces the distress to the family of the deceased, prevents delay and reflects the common law duty on everyone to report a death to a coroner if it occurred in circumstances that might give rise to an inquest (*R v Clark* [1702]; *R v Wiltshire Coroner ex p. Clegg* (1996)). In a review of the death registration and coroner system, it was found that only some 3.4% of cases are reported to the coroner by the registrar (Home Office, 2003). Once the doctor has reported the

---

Box 10.1 Regulation 41 of the Births and Death Regulations (1987)

This regulation requires a Registrar to report a death to the coroner if the death is one:

a. in respect of which the deceased was not attended during his last illness by a registered medical practitioner; or
b. in respect of which the registrar:

   i. has been unable to obtain a duly completed certificate of cause of death; or

   ii. has received such a certificate with respect to which it appears to him, from the particulars contained in the certificate or otherwise that the deceased was not seen by the certifying medical practitioner either after death or within 14 days before death; or
c. the cause of which appears to be unknown; or
d. which the registrar has reason to believe to have been unnatural or to have been caused by violence or neglect or by abortion or to have been attended by suspicious circumstances; or
e. which appears to the registrar to have occurred during an operation or before recovery from the effect of an anaesthetic; or
f. which appears to the registrar from the contents of any medical certificate of cause of death to have been due to industrial disease or industrial poisoning

(Crown Copyright material is reproduced with the permission of the Controller of HMSO and the Queen's Printer for Scotland)

---

death to the coroner, a number of outcomes are possible, as seen in Fig. 10.1.

If the doctor is qualified to complete the medical certificate, i.e. the doctor attended the patient during his or her last illness, saw the patient within 14 days of death or the body after death and is confident about the cause of death, then the matter may be discussed informally with the coroner and the certificate of cause of death completed and initialled on the back stating that the matter has been discussed with the coroner.

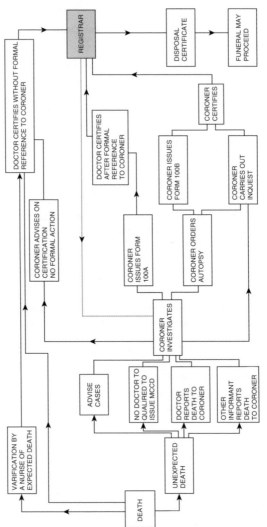

Fig 10.1 The process of registering a death.

If the doctor is not qualified under the Births and Deaths Regulations 1987 to complete the certificate, the matter can still be discussed with the coroner, who may decide that no action is necessary and a form 100A will be issued (no inquest or post-mortem necessary) to the registrar.

If the cause of death is unknown, the coroner is very likely to ask for a post-mortem. If this confirms the cause of death as natural causes it is open to the coroner to issue pink form B (form 100), no inquest following post-mortem, to the registrar as even though the death was sudden the cause is now known and does not warrant an inquest.

The coroner may decide after considering the post-mortem report and circumstances of the death to hold an inquest. If the cause of death is unnatural, the coroner may be obliged to hold an inquest. Until this has been completed, the patient's death will not be registered, but the coroner will be able to release the body for the funeral soon after the cause of death is known and issue an order for burial or certificate for cremation (Coroners Rules, 1984, r. 60). After the inquest the coroner will issue a certificate after inquest, stating the cause of death, to the registrar to allow the death to be registered. The process of holding an inquest is discussed in detail in Chapter 12.

With knowledge of the administrative system for registering a death, nurses can reassure and support the patient's family through the process that frequently adds to the distress caused by the death of a loved one.

REQUIREMENTS FOR VERIFICATION BY NURSES OF EXPECTED DEATH

Verification of death is a procedure for determining whether a person has actually died. All deaths must be subject to professional verification that life has ended (Home Office, 2003). This is different from the certification process and can be performed by a medical practitioner or by any other suitable qualified professional, for example a registered nurse.

In many areas, nurses are entitled, under protocol, to verify the death of a patient in cases of expected death. This facilitates the timely removal of the body to a recognised chapel of rest within the coroner's district and the medical certificate of cause of death is issued later by the patient's last attending doctor (Ayris, 2002). The coroner generally agrees the protocol or policy through a memorandum of understanding that must be followed.

An expected death is defined as one where both the patient's demise is anticipated in the near future and the doctor will be able to issue a medical certificate of the cause of death (i.e. the doctor will have seen the patient within the last 14 days before the death). The patient's doctor should indicate in the records that the patient's condition is life-threatening and death is expected.

A nurse would not, therefore, be entitled to verify death where:

- Death is sudden or unexpected, for example in hospital this would include a death that has occurred within 24 h of admission, where no firm clinical diagnosis has been made.
- In cases of expected death, the death occurs in an unexpected manner or in unexpected circumstances.
- Death has occurred as a result of an untoward incident such as a fall or medication error.

A nurse entitled to verify death following a protocol will conduct an examination that reflects the requirements of Triad of Bichat, i.e. they will verify that:

- There is no response to painful stimuli, determined by sternal rub for 10 s.
- There is an absence of carotid pulse after palpation for 1 min.
- There is an absence of heart sounds, determined by stethoscope, after a minimum of 1 min.
- There is an absence of respiratory activity, determined by observation and assessment with stethoscope, after a minimum of 1 min.
- There are fixed, dilated pupils that do not react to light, determined by shining a torch light into the patient's eye and observing for any change in shape or size, and repeated in each eye.

The results of the observations must be recorded in the patient's notes together with details of any equipment removed and the amount of any medication remaining at the time of death. The nurse verifying the death must sign his or her name, status and date and time of carrying out the procedure (Ayris, 2002).

Where the verification procedure requires the nurse to pass on news of a death to family, it is essential that this is done with care, sensitivity and accuracy. Giving distressing and inaccurate information can give rise to liability in negligence. In *Allin v City and Hackney HA* [1996], a mother successfully sued for the post-traumatic stress she suffered as a result of being mistakenly told by a nurse that her child had died.

STATUS OF THE BODY AFTER DEATH

Body as property

Unlike houses or other buildings and smaller possessions that can be bequeathed in a will, our bodies do not have the status of property and cannot be passed on by way of gift. No other rule of law can claim as macabre a passage through history as the legal rule that there is 'no property in a corpse'. It is an area of law where slavers, grave robbers, grieving widows, freak show exhibitors and harvesters of body parts have featured prominently.

This odd common law rule developed from *R v Haynes* (1614). *Haynes* was indicted for stealing the winding sheets that were wrapped around dead bodies. The court held that a corpse could not own property (the winding sheet) but this was later misread as there being no property in a corpse. This interpretation has persisted at common law for over 150 years in cases such as *Bourne v Norwich Crematorium Ltd* [1967], where the local inspector of taxes denied tax relief on a new crematorium chimney stack as it was not processing goods.

More recently, the Court of Appeal confirmed the rule in *R v Kelly* [1998], where Lord Justice Rose held that, however questionable the origins of the principle, only parliament could change it now because of its long history. The implication of the rule is that little or no heed need be taken of the wishes of the deceased in terms of disposing of the body after death. For example, in *Williams v Williams* (1882), the deceased left instructions in his will that the executors should allow a woman named in the will to cremate his body. The executors disregarded these instructions and buried the deceased. The court held that the right of disposal rests solely with the executors and it was for them to decide how it was done.

An exception for work and skill

An exception to the general rule that there is no property in a corpse exists in cases where the body or body parts have been subjected to work or skill that has resulted in the body acquiring attributes differentiating it from a 'mere corpse' (*Doodewood v Spence* (1908)).

In *R v Kelly* [1998], an artist was convicted of theft along with an accomplice who had removed body parts from the Royal College of Surgeons. Kelly argued that body parts could not be stolen as they were not property, but the Court of Appeal held that as work and skill had been applied in preserving the body parts they had become property and Kelly was guilty of theft.

Methods of disposal
Burial

Historically, the method of disposal of a human body after death has been by means of burial (*Kemp v Wickes* (1809)). To this day, every inhabitant of a parish and every person dying within the parish has a common law right to be buried in the parish burial ground (*Hughes v Lloyd* (1888)).

The other main method of disposal is cremation. This has been lawful since the late 19th century when the case of *R v Price* (1884) held that cremation was not unlawful provided the burning was done in such a manner as not to cause a nuisance. Nowadays, the place, manner and conditions of cremation are regulated by the Cremation Acts of 1902 and 1952. It is an offence to effect any cremation outside the provisions of these statutes. A person does not have a legal right to be cremated.

Cremation

For a cremation to take place, the deceased's personal representative must submit a statutory application completed by two doctors, which is then checked by a medical referee at the crematorium who decides on final approval (Cremation Act, 1902). If the deceased's case is reported to the coroner for inquest then the coroner must issue a cremation certificate instead (Coroners Act, 1988).

Although cremation and burial are the common means of disposal, other methods are not forbidden. For example, in *R v*

Dudley & Stevens (1884), sailors who ate the flesh of a dead ship-mate to survive a shipwreck had not committed any crime. Disposing of a body by eating would therefore not be unlawful. Other examples include the plastic lamination of a body and the freezing of a body or the head and brain of the deceased. The Public Health (Control of Diseases) Act, 1984 also allows the Secretary of State for Health to create regulations for alternative methods of disposal where they feel this is necessary.

Right of disposal of a body

The 'no property in a corpse' rule severely restricts the deceased's ability to direct the method of disposal of their body. A method that might be used to overcome this limitation is by way of con-ditional gift, i.e. a gift in the deceased's will that is made on condition that the wishes of testator are carried out. For example, Frances Power Cobbe had a dread of being buried alive. She made a conditional gift in her will of some 50 guineas to the executor if the executor brought a surgeon to her funeral, with a similar amount to the surgeon if he severed her throat with a scalpel just before she was interred to make sure she was dead.

The main drawback of a gift is that it can be declined. Lord Avebury, liberal peer and Buddhist, gifted his body to science for dissection and the remains to Battersea dogs' home as dog food. This part of the gift was declined.

Duty of disposal

While maintaining the 'no property in a corpse' rule, the law recognises that there is a duty on certain individuals to arrange for the disposal of the deceased. The law accepts that to discharge this duty, the individual has the right to lawful possession of the body.

In health care the concept of the next of kin is usually relied on to identify the patient's closest relative. In relation to the law of death, the hierarchy of entitlement to lawful possession of the body does not place the next of kin first. The person with greatest claim to lawful possession of the body is the executor of the deceased's will, who can decide on the method of disposal even where the deceased has left instructions to the contrary (*Williams v Williams* (1882)).

The close relatives of the deceased do not have a greater claim to lawful possession than the executor. In *Rees v Hughes* [1946], the court of appeal held that the duty to bury a wife is that of her executor, not her husband. Similarly in *Grandison v Nembhard* (1989), a daughter objected to her father being buried back in his native Jamaica. The court held that the executor was entitled to dispose of the deceased's body and had discretion as to the mode and place of disposal. The court would not interfere with the exercise of the discretion unless the executor had acted unreasonably. Neither the distress nor the inconvenience to his daughter nor the extra expense involved would justify the court's interference.

Where the deceased has died intestate, i.e. without making a will, the person authorised to administer the estate is entitled to lawful possession. In *Holtham v Arnold* (1986), Charles Arnold died intestate at St Bartholomew's Hospital. At that time he had been living for two years with Alice Holtham, who made arrangements for his burial in accordance with his verbal wishes. His wife, however, wanted him to be cremated and instructed the hospital not to release his body. The court held that Mrs Arnold, being entitled to letters of administration of her husband's estate, was also entitled to lawful possession of his corpse in order to dispose of it. The court further held that had the deceased made a will appointing Miss Holtham his executor, then she would have been entitled to arrange the funeral.

Where there is no executor or administrator of the deceased's estate, the court has placed the duty of disposal on:

- The owner of the property where the person died (*R v Feist* (1858)), for example where a patient without relatives or funds died in a hospital or care, the managers of the hospital or the care home would have the duty to arrange and pay for the funeral.
- The parents of an unmarried child: In *R v Gwynedd County Council ex p B* (1991) a looked-after child died in the care of the local authority who wanted to arrange the funeral. The court held that once the child died, responsibility for the child's body returned to the parents, who were entitled to lawful possession, to arrange the funeral.

- Other surviving relatives are entitled to administer the estate under The Non-Contentious Probate Rules, 1987.
- The local authority where the body lies: The Public Health (Control of Diseases) Act 1984, section 46(1) provides that it is the duty of every local authority to cremate or bury a person who has died or been found dead in their area where it appears that no suitable arrangements have been made for the disposal of the body. The authority is entitled to recover its expenses from the deceased's estate or spouse or parent if they can be found. For example, a child found dead in a river in Devon was buried a year later by the local authority when an investigation to trace her parents failed (Horton, 2003).

On the death of a patient in a hospital or care home, the Trust managing the hospital or the owners of the care home will be in lawful possession of the body until a person with greater entitlement in the hierarchy, such as a close relative or executor of the person's will, seeks lawful possession. Lawful possession of the body gives rise to a duty to ensure that any property on or with the deceased is properly accounted for and safeguarded until it can be passed on to the patient's representative.

Evidential certainty demands that an accurate written record of any property remaining on the body or kept in safe keeping is properly completed and each stage of a transfer of property is signed and receipted in order to avoid liability.

ORGAN DONATION

The Human Tissue Act 2004 put in place a legal framework to modernise the law in relation to human tissue and organs. It regulates the removal, storage and use of human tissue, and repeals and replaces the Human Tissue Act 1961, the Anatomy Act 1984 and the Human Organ Transplants Act 1989.

The Human Tissue Act 2004 regulates the storage and use of whole bodies and the removal, storage and use of relevant material from the body of a deceased person (Human Tissue Act 2004, section 1). Relevant material is any material consisting of, or including, human cells. The exceptions are gametes and embryos outside the body, and hair and nail from a living person (unless the purpose is to analyse DNA). The definition therefore includes materials such as blood, bone marrow, skin, kidneys and other human tissue.

The key principle underpinning the lawful use or retention of human body parts, organs and tissue is consent. Valid consent from an appropriate person, known as an appropriate consent, is required for an activity regulated by the act to be lawful (see Box 10.2).

Box 10.2 Uses of human tissue requiring consent under the Human Tissue Act 2004. Source: Human Tissue Act 2004, schedule 1, parts 1 & 2

Part 1:

Purposes requiring consent: living and deceased

- Anatomical examination.
- Determining the cause of death.
- Establishing after a person's death the efficacy of any drug or other treatment administered to him.
- Obtaining scientific or medical information about a living or deceased person, which may be relevant to any other person (including a future person).
- Public display.
- Research in connection with disorders or the functioning of the human body.
- Transplantation.

Part 2:

Purposes requiring consent: deceased persons

- Clinical audit.
- Education or training relating to human health.
- Performance assessment.
- Public health monitoring.
- Quality assurance.

(Crown Copyright material is reproduced with the permission of the Controller of HMSO and the Queen's Printer for Scotland)

As a further safeguard, storing a body for anatomical examination and the examination itself may only lawfully proceed where:

- There is an appropriate consent that is in writing and witnessed before death.
- The death has been registered under the appropriate births and deaths registration statute.

The Act provides for some exemptions to this requirement, such as where a post mortem is required by a coroner (see Box 10.3).

Appropriate consent

The Human Tissue Act 2004 makes an appropriate consent the underpinning principle for the lawfulness of activities regulated by the Act. To be valid the consent must be obtained from an appropriate person and given in accordance with the requirements of the Act and its code of practice (Human Tissue Act 2004, section 1). For example, if a body is to be used for anatomical examination or public display, then only the consent of the person in writing and witnessed before their death is accepted as an appropriate consent (Human Tissue Act 2004, sections 2 and 3).

Box 10.3 Exemptions to the general requirement for an appropriate consent

- Existing holdings: Human tissue already held in storage prior to April 2006.
- Imported tissue: Tissue that has been imported or taken from a body that has been imported or comes from a person who died at least 100 years before the need for consent came into force.
- Coroner: Exemption for anything done for purposes of functions of a coroner or under the authority of a coroner.

(Crown Copyright material is reproduced with the permission of the Controller of HMSO and the Queen's Printer for Scotland)

Appropriate consent for children

Given the furore following the public inquiry into the retention of organs at Liverpool Children's Hospital, the Act makes specific provision for appropriate consent in relation to children.

Living children who are competent to do so may give their own consent. If they are not competent or choose not to make a decision then appropriate consent can be taken from a person with parental responsibility for them. Competence is not defined in the Act and hence will be established by the rule in *Gillick v West Norfolk and Wisbech AHA* [1986] for children under 16 and by the Family Law Reform Act 1969, (section 8) for those who are 16–18 years (Human Tissue Act 2004, section 2). A competent child may also make an advanced decision to give or refuse consent under the 2004 Act, and where this is valid and applicable, it will have effect.

Where nurses consider children to have sufficient maturity and intelligence to be capable of making such a decision in relation to the use of their tissue or organs, their consent will be valid. If a child refuses permission then that refusal must be respected.

The consent of a competent child to have their body used for anatomical examination or public display must be in writing and witnessed. No one other than a competent child may give consent to the use of their body for the purposes of anatomical examination or public display. Where a child has not dealt with the issue of consent for one of the other purposes regulated by the Human Tissue Act 2004 the consent of someone with parental responsibility will be the appropriate consent.

Appropriate consent for adults

The Human Tissue Act 2004 also sets out the meaning of appropriate consent in relation to activities concerning the body of a deceased adult or relevant material from a person who is at the time of the activity a living or deceased adult.

If the adult is alive then the adult must give consent (Human Tissue Act 2004, section 3). After death, the written and witnessed consent of the adult is required in advance for the purpose of anatomical examination or public display. This may be in the form of a separate document or in a duly completed will (Wills Act 1837, section 9). For other scheduled purposes under the Act and where there is no prior decision, a person nominated by the adult to make such decisions after death may give consent.

Adults can appoint one or more nominated representatives who may give consent after their death to storage or use of their body, or removal, storage and use of relevant material from their body for scheduled purposes. This may be made:

- Orally before two witnesses.
- In writing by the person or on the person's behalf and attested by one witness.
- Made in a valid will.

Where two or more people are appointed they will be assumed to be able to act alone unless the appointment says they must act together.

The Human Tissue Act 2004 introduces a fundamental change in the law relating to the use of human tissue, body parts and organs. Contrary to the long-established 'no property in a corpse' rule, a person can now state that he or she wishes to donate body parts or tissue after death, and health professionals will have to respect that wish.

The wishes of the deceased will now take precedence over the relatives' wishes or the person in lawful possession of the body such as the executor of a will. The Human Tissue Act 2004 gives priority to the wishes of the 13.5 million people on the NHS organ donor register and to those who have made it clear that they would like their organs to be donated in the event of their death. To allow for the wishes of the deceased to become known to the transplant authorities, the Act allows for the steps to be taken, such as cold perfusion, i.e. to preserve the organs following death (Human Tissue Act 2004, section 43).

Health professionals, including nurses, have an important role in advising patients about the consent requirements of the Act, how to make their wishes known and how to lawfully nominate a representative who can carry out their wishes after their death.

Human Tissue Authority

To ensure that the rights of individuals subject to the activities regulated by the Human Tissue Act 2004 are paramount, the Act established a Human Tissue Authority to oversee and provide guidance on compliance. The Authority has a general role in informing the public and the Secretary of State for Health about such issues as the:

- Storage and use of human bodies and tissue.
- Removal of tissue from human bodies for scheduled purposes.
- Import and export of bodies and human tissue for scheduled purposes.
- Disposal of human tissue, including imported tissue, following its use in medical treatment or for scheduled purposes.

The Authority has issued codes of practice covering consent, communicating with relatives regarding post mortems, anatomical examination, import and export, existing holdings and disposal of tissue (Human Tissue Authority, 2006).

The Authority also licenses a number of activities and carries out inspections to ensure compliance with the Act in relation to the:

- Storage and use of human bodies for anatomical examination and related research.
- Conducting of post-mortem examinations, including removal and retention of human tissue.
- Removal of human tissue from the body of a deceased person for other scheduled purposes, except transplantation.
- Storage and use of human bodies or parts for public display.
- Storage of human tissue for other scheduled purposes, for example human tissue banking for transplant purposes or research under the EC Tissues and Cells Directive (2004/23/EC).

LAW RELATING TO LIFE-SUSTAINING TREATMENT

The development of the law relating to life-sustaining treatment has focused on three key areas:

- The duty to provide treatment.
- The extent of patient autonomy in relation to the right to refuse life-sustaining treatment or to require more direct methods of ending life such as euthanasia or assisted dying.

- The health professional's right to withhold or withdraw treatment.

For example, in *R (adult: medical treatment)* [1996], a psychiatrist was concerned that another admission to hospital would not be in the best interests of a 23-year-old man born with a malformation of the brain and cerebral palsy. The psychiatrist signed a direction headed 'do not resuscitate', which was challenged on the patient's behalf. The court held that a 'do not resuscitate' policy may be appropriate where CPR was unlikely to be successful. The court recognised that two areas of law had to be considered and carefully weighed before arriving at a decision not to resuscitate a patient.

Duty to provide treatment

The duty of care to the patient that includes a duty to provide treatment has to be weighed against the principle that there is no duty to provide treatment where doing so would be futile (*Airedale NHS Trust v Bland* [1993]).

In *Airedale NHS Trust v Bland* [1993], the House of Lords held that when a person, whether they be a health professional such as a nurse or a relative or friend, undertakes to care for an individual, they owe a duty to that person to care for them appropriately and not cause harm. A breach of that duty can result in both criminal and civil liability.

In *R v Stone & Dobinson* [1977], a couple took in Stone's ageing anorexic sister who was found dead some six months later covered in pressure sores and emaciated in a soiled bed. The Court of Appeal held that on taking the sister into their home, the couple had undertaken a duty to care for her, which they had breached. They were each sentenced to 18 months' imprisonment for manslaughter.

In *R(Burke) v GMC* [2005], the Court of Appeal held that once a patient is accepted in to hospital, the health staff come under a positive duty to care for the patient. A fundamental aspect of this is a duty to take such steps as are reasonable to keep the patient alive.

Nurses would normally be required to provide life-sustaining treatment to patients in their care who required it.

Patient autonomy

The duty to provide treatment imposed on health professionals, such as nurses, when they undertake to care for a patient does not, however, allow them to override the wishes of a capable adult patient.

A capable adult is entitled to refuse treatment even where this would lead to their death (*Re MB (Caesarean Section)* [1997]). In *R v Smith* [1979], the court ordered that a man be found not guilty of the manslaughter of his wife who died when he accepted her wish not to call for an ambulance or medical assistance when complications arose during a home confinement. The judge directed that the woman was a capable adult whose valid refusal of care absolved her husband of his duty towards her.

Similarly, where a capable adult patient requests that no life-sustaining treatment be given then that wish must be respected. The wish may be put in an advance decision refusing treatment that will come into effect when the person is incapable (Mental Capacity Act 2005, section 24).

Advance decisions refusing treatment

To be a valid advanced decision, the patient must have been a capable adult at the time of making the decision and it should not contain a request for an action that would be unlawful, such as active euthanasia.

Where an advance decision refusing treatment concerns the refusal of life-sustaining treatment, the Mental Capacity Act 2005 requires that the decision:

- Be made in writing either by the person or written on their behalf.
- Be signed by the maker or signed on their behalf in their presence.
- Be witnessed in writing in the presence of the maker.
- Contains a statement verifying that it is to apply 'even if life is at risk'.

However, an advance decision cannot be used to ask for anything that is illegal, such as euthanasia or for help to commit suicide. Nor can it refuse the offer of food and drink by mouth or measures solely designed to maintain comfort, such as providing appropriate pain relief, warmth or shelter and basic nursing care essential for comfort, such as washing, bathing and mouth care.

Proxy refusal of life-sustaining treatment

As well as a person's ability to have his or her wishes regarding life-sustaining treatment respected through advance decisions refusing treatment, the Mental Capacity Act 2005 also allows a capable adult to nominate others to make personal welfare decisions, should he or she become incapable, through a 'personal welfare lasting power of attorney'.

Personal welfare includes consenting to or refusing medical treatment and the Mental Capacity Act 2005, section 11, allows people to give their attorney the right to refuse life-sustaining treatment on their behalf. This right only comes into force where the lasting power of attorney has been registered with the public guardian and the person, now called the donor, is incapable.

Where a person with power to make decisions regarding life-sustaining treatment on behalf of an incapable adult refuses such treatment, nurses are bound by that decision as if it were the patient who was refusing it.

No right to demand treatment

While autonomy and self-determination allow a capable adult patient to refuse treatment, even if it leads to death, it does not allow a person to demand a specific form of health care.

The legal obligation to provide treatment is not based on a patient demanding a particular form of treatment. The treatment a patient receives and is asked to consent to is based on the clinical need of the patient and the nurse's obligation to provide that treatment as part of the duty of care.

No requirement to provide futile treatment

For incapable adults who have not made their wishes known through an advance decision refusing treatment, the law holds that whilst there is a very strong presumption in favour of taking steps that would prolong life, the obligation is not absolute (*R (Burke) v GMC & Others* [2004]).

Nurses are not required to continue giving treatment or to intervene when doing so would be futile and prolong the

---

Box 10.4 Definition of serious medical treatment.
Source: Mental Capacity Act 2005 (independent mental capacity advocates) (general) Regulations 2006 (SI 2006/1832)

Serious medical treatment is treatment that involves providing, withdrawing or withholding treatment in circumstances where:

- In a case where a single treatment is being proposed, there is a fine balance between its benefits to the patient and the burdens and risks it is likely to entail for him.
- In a case where there is a choice of treatments, a decision as to which one to use is finely balanced.
- What is proposed would be likely to involve serious consequences for the patient.

(Crown Copyright material is reproduced with the permission of the Controller of HMSO and the Queen's Printer for Scotland)

---

suffering of the person concerned (*Airedale NHS Trust v Bland* [1993]). As important as the sanctity of life is, it may have to take second place to human dignity.

The Mental Capacity Act 2005, section 4, requires that best interests be determined according to a statutory checklist of factors that includes the ascertainable wishes of the person and consultation with one or more persons interested in the care of the person. Where the incapable adult is unbefriended and there is no one to consult, it is necessary to instruct an independent mental capacity advocate to review the case before a life-sustaining treatment can be withheld or withdrawn.

Withholding or withdrawing life-sustaining treatment meets the definition of serious medical treatment that triggers a duty to instruct an independent advocate under the 2005 Act (see Box 10.4).

EUTHANASIA

The term 'euthanasia' is derived from the Greek meaning 'easy death' or 'dying well'. This broad definition adds to the confusion over the contemporary meaning of the word. It is difficult to argue that a person should not be entitled to an 'easy death' and this is the basis of palliative care in the UK. Nurses in palliative care would rightly argue that this does not equate to euthanasia.

Definitions

A more realistic definition would be the process whereby life is ended by another to avoid the distressing effects of an illness (Kennedy & Grubb, 1998).

Mason and McCall Smith (1994) have further classified euthanasia as:

- *Voluntary:* where the person killed either requests death or agrees to it.
- *Non-voluntary:* where it is considered to be in the person's best interest to end his or her life because of intractable pain or suffering but where the person is incapable of expressing his or her own view and so a proxy is used to request that the life be ended.
- *Involuntary:* where the person killed either objects or cannot express an opinion and has not given advanced permission.

Each of these classifications may be:

- *Active:* where a deliberate act terminates life, such as giving a lethal injection of a drug.
- *Passive:* where treatment that would keep the person alive is withheld or withdrawn.

Active euthanasia

Active euthanasia is a process where the death of a person results from a specific act directed at causing the death. The intention of the person carrying out the act must be that the person will die (Kennedy & Grubb, 1998). An intention to relieve suffering by giving sedation and analgesia whose secondary effects are to shorten life is not considered active euthanasia and is lawful under the principle of double effect (*Airedale NHS Trust v Bland* [1993]).

Active euthanasia is not currently tolerated and the position of the law has changed little since the case of *R v Bodkin Adams* [1957], where the judge said at 366:

'If the acts done are intended to kill and do kill it does not matter
if a life is cut short by weeks or months, it is just as much murder
as if it were cut short by years.'

This is the case, regardless of whether people voluntarily
request an end to their suffering or a nurse decides that it is in
the best interests of the patient to end their suffering by killing
them.

In *R v Cox* (1992), a consultant rheumatologist promised a
patient that he would not allow her to suffer as the result of her
incurable illness. She reminded him of his promise when in considerable and intractable pain, and Dr Cox gave her a lethal dose
of potassium chloride. Details of the incident did not emerge until
after the funeral and as there was no corroborating evidence, the
doctor was convicted of attempted murder.

Involuntary active euthanasia is a concept most groups press-
ing for a change in the law are eager to distance themselves from
(Kennedy & Grubb, 1998). It involves ending patients' lives
without their personal or proxy invitation to do so. Although the
motivation to act is based on a desire to relieve suffering, it is the
paternalistic decision as to what is best for a person that causes
concern and is a warning against giving health professionals
unfettered powers over life and death.

In *R v Carr* [1986], a doctor gave a patient suffering from the
latter stages of lung cancer a lethal dose of phenobarbitone. In
his summing up, Justice Mars-Jones held that:

'However gravely ill a man may be he is entitled in our law to
every hour that God has granted him. That hour may be the most
precious and important of his life.'

This was precisely the concern raised by the relatives of a patient
subject to a lethal injection by a nurse. The nurse gave a lethal
25 mg dose of Nozinan to the 79-year-old patient as in her view
he should not be suffering but going to heaven. She gave the drug
without authority and against advice in the patient's medical
notes, for although the patient was suffering from lymphoma his
current condition was due to pneumonia and he was responding
to treatment. In an echo of Justice Mars-Jones' sentiments, the
patient's relatives stated that the nurse had stolen the chance to

say goodbye to their father from them and that had caused considerable hurt (Horsnell, 2007).

Similarly, in *R v Salisbury* [2005], a ward sister was convicted of the attempted murder of two of her patients after the jury heard evidence that she had administered high doses of diamorphine and was overheard telling a patient to 'give in, it is time to go'. The Court of Appeal accepted that the ward sister had administered controlled drugs to her patients with the intention of killing them and had been motivated by a desire to free up beds. She received a five-year jail term.

Both voluntary and involuntary forms of active euthanasia are prohibited under the law in the UK. A person who deliberately acts to end the suffering of others by killing them would be charged with murder, attempted murder or manslaughter, depending on circumstances of the case. Health professionals would also face further censure from the regulatory bodies.

Passive euthanasia

Passive euthanasia is distinguished from active euthanasia as the means of ending life is not by the use of a direct action such as a lethal injection of drugs but by withholding treatment and care necessary to keep the person alive, for example refusing to treat an infection in a terminally ill person in the hope that the untreated infection will lead to the person's death and bring an end to their suffering.

Steinbock (1980) argues that active and passive euthanasia are indistinguishable, as omitting to treat is as potent as actively killing a person. In his view, there is no difference between giving a lethal injection and omitting antibiotics for an infection if the intention is that the person should die as a result.

In law, however, there is a real distinction in culpability where a death occurs as a result of an action by a third person compared to a death resulting from a person omitting to act. We are all protected in law from harmful acts but criminal liability for harm that results from a failure to act is reserved for circumstances where a duty to act arises. For example, in *R v Instan* [1893], a woman undertook to care for her aunt but when the aunt became ill and was unable to feed herself or call medical advice, the niece stood by refusing to feed her or call for help. *Instan* was convicted of manslaughter.

In *Airedale NHS Trust v Bland* [1993], the House of Lords recognised the concept of medical futility and held that it would be lawful to withhold treatment, in this case artificial nutrition and hydration from a man in a persistent vegetative state, where it was no longer in the patient's best interests to continue with that treatment. Lord Mustill sums up the position in this way:

'The cessation of nourishment and hydration is an omission not an act.'

Accordingly, the cessation will not be a criminal act unless the doctors are under a present duty to continue the regime'

At the time when Anthony Bland came into the care of the doctors, decisions had to be made about his care, which he was unable to make for himself. These decisions were to be made in his best interests. Since the possibility that he might recover still existed, his best interests required that he should be supported in the hope that this would happen. All hope of recovery has now been abandoned. Thus, although the termination of his life is not in the best interests of Anthony Bland, his best interests in continuing with the treatment have also disappeared.

Since there is no longer a duty to provide nourishment and hydration, a failure to do so cannot be a criminal offence. Where continuing with treatment is futile, the duty to provide that treatment ceases and it is not a crime to withhold it. However, an omission to treat cannot be justified on the grounds that it would be in the best interests of the patient to die. Indeed, the courts have consistently restated their view that it can never be in a person's best interests to die (*Burke v GMC & others* [2005]). Even under statute law, a determination of a person's best interests cannot be motivated by a desire to bring about a person's death (Mental Capacity Act 2005, section 4(5)).

In *Burke v GMC & others* [2005], a man was concerned that the artificial nutrition required to keep him alive would be withdrawn when it was still of benefit to him and he would suffer as the result of slowly dying from thirst and starvation. He challenged the lawfulness of the General Medical Council's guidance on withholding treatment and made it clear in an advanced statement that he wanted to be kept alive by artificial means. The Court of Appeal held that:

> 'It seems to us that for a doctor deliberately to interrupt life-prolonging treatment in the face of a patient's expressed wish to be kept alive, with the intention of thereby terminating the patient's life, would leave the doctor with no answer to a charge of murder.'
>
> *(Burke v GMC & others* [2005],
> Lord Phillips at paragraph 34)

To terminate a person's life by passive means, such as withholding life-sustaining treatment or denying the person treatment for an infection when there continues to be a positive duty to care for the patient is unlawful. Nurses cannot make a determination of patients' best interests on the basis that they are better off dead. Any withholding or withdrawing of treatment must be on the grounds that such treatment is futile and of no benefit to the patient (*Airedale NHS Trust v Bland* [1993]).

It is clear from the cases of *R v Cox* (1992), *Airedale NHS Trust v Bland* [1993] and *Burke v GMC & others* [2005] that both active and passive euthanasia is unlawful in the UK. Any nurse who deliberately ends the life of a patient to relieve their suffering by either active or passive means would be liable to a charge of murder.

Assisted dying

A possible middle ground in the euthanasia debate is the notion of assisted dying or assisted suicide. Rather than a person being killed by another to end their suffering, they are given the means to end their own lives when they feel they can no longer go on living with their condition.

This form of intervention is also prohibited in law by the Suicide Act 1961. Although it is no longer an offence to take one's own life (Suicide Act 1961, section 1), it remains an offence to 'aid, abet, counsel or procure the suicide of another or an attempt by another to commit suicide' (Suicide Act 1961, s 2(1)). Assisted suicide is prohibited whether performed by a relative, friend or a nurse, and a person who does so would be liable on conviction to 14 years in prison.

The aim of the prohibition is to protect vulnerable people from being pressured into killing themselves by unscrupulous family or friends. In *R v McShane* [1977], a daughter was found guilty of trying to persuade her 89-year-old mother, who was residing in a nursing home, to kill herself so that she could inherit her mother's estate. The police obtained incriminating evidence of the daughter by using a hidden camera at the nursing home that showed the daughter handing her mother drugs, hidden in a packet of sweets, and pinning a note on her mother's dress telling her not to 'bungle it'!

The same provisions also prevent people who cannot take their own lives because of a debilitating condition from being helped to do so by a friend, relative or nurse. In *Pretty v DPP* [2001], the House of Lords refused to grant Diane Pretty's application for a judicial review challenging the decision of the Director of Public Prosecutions, who had refused to give an undertaking that he would not prosecute her husband if he assisted in her suicide at some time in the future.

The European Court of Human Rights subsequently confirmed that the Suicide Act 1961 did not violate the European Convention on Human Rights as:

- The right to life protected under Article 2 did not include a right to die at a chosen time.
- It was not the government subjecting Mrs Pretty to inhuman or degrading treatment under Article 3 but the motor neurone disease from which she suffered.
- Mrs Pretty's right to respect for her private life under Article 8 was not absolute. The right could be restricted by the government passing legislation, which had the legitimate aim of protecting vulnerable individuals from being forced into agreeing to be assisted to die.
- Banning assisted suicide, therefore, was not a disproportionate or unlawful action by the government.

Aiding, abetting, counselling or procuring a person's suicide is therefore unlawful even though a patient's own act of suicide is not criminal. A nurse who intended to assist a patient to take their own life by providing them with a bottle of potentially lethal tablets could face a charge under the Suicide Act 1961, section 2, and face up to 14 years in prison.

CONCLUSION

In this chapter, an overview of the legal issues of death has been detailed. A definition of death has been discussed. The process of certification and registration of death, together with the process for reporting a death to the coroner, have been described. The requirements for verification by nurses of expected death have been stated and the status of the body after death has been outlined. The issues associated with organ donation, life-sustaining treatment and euthanasia have been discussed.

REFERENCES

Airedale NHS Trust v Bland [1993] AC 789.

Allin v City and Hackney HA [1996] 7 Med LR 167.

Ayris WW (2002) Verification of expected death by district nurses. *Br J Community Nurs* 7(7): 370.

Bourne v Norwich Crematorium Ltd [1967] 1 WLR 691.

Burke v GMC & others [2005] EWCA Civ 1003 ((CA).

Coroners Rules 1984 (SI 1984/552).

Doodewood v Spence (1908) 6 CLR 406.

Gillick v West Norfolk and Wisbech AHA [1986] AC 112 ((HL)).

Grandison v Nembhard (1989) 4 BMLR 140.

Holtham v Arnold (1986) 2 BMLR 123.

Home Office (2003) Death Certification and Investigation in England, Wales and Northern Ireland. The Report of a Fundamental Review (Cmd 5831). TSO, London.

Horsnell M (2007) Nurse gave patient fatal drug dose to help him pass over. (news item), *The Times*, 8 March, p. 8.

Horton G (2003) Abandoned baby girl will not be forgotten. (news item), *Western Morning News* p. 33.

Hughes v Lloyd (1888) 2 QBD 157.

Human Tissue Authority (2006) Code of Practice – Consent Code 1. HTA, London.

Kemp v Wickes (1809) 3 Phillim 264.

Kennedy I, Grubb A (1998) *Principles of Medical Law*. OUP, Oxford.

Mason JK, McCall Smith RA (1994) *Law and Medical Ethics*. Butterworth, London.

Pretty v DPP [2001] UKHL 61.

R (adult: medical treatment) [1996] 2 FLR 99.

R (Burke) v GMC & others [2004] EWHC 1879 (Admin).

R v Bodkin Adams [1957] Crim LR 365.

R v Carr [1986] *Times Law Report* 30th November pge 1.

R v Clark [1702] 1 Salk 377.

R v Cox (1992) 12 BMLR 38.

R v Dudley & Stevens (1884) 14 QBD 273.

R v Feist (1858) Dears & B 590.

R v Gwynedd County Council ex p B (1991) 7 BMLR 120.

R v Haynes (1614) 12 Co.Rep 113.

R v Instan [1893] 1 QB 450.

R v Kelly [1998] 3 All ER 741.

R v Malcherek & Steel [1981] 1 WLR 690.

R v McShane [1977] Crim LR 737.

R v Price (1884) 12 QBD 247.

R v Salisbury [2005] EWCA Crim 3107 (CA).

R v Smith [1979] Crim LR 251.

R v Stone & Dobinson [1977] QB 354.

R v Wiltshire Coroner ex p. Clegg (1996) 161 JP 521.

R(Burke) v GMC [2005] EWCA 1003.

Re A (1992) 3 Med LR 303 (CA).

Re MB (Caesarean Section) [1997] 2 F.L.R. 426.

Rees v Hughes [1946] KB 517.

Steinbock B (1980) *Killing and Letting Die*. Prentice Hall, New Jersey.

The Non-Contentious Probate Rules 1987 (SI 1987/2024)

The Shipman Inquiry (2004) *Fifth Report: Safeguarding Patients: Lessons from the Past – Proposals for the Future (Cm 6394)*. The Stationery Office, London.

Williams v Williams (1882) 20 Ch D 659.

Post Mortems and Inquests | 11

Cassam Tengnah

INTRODUCTION

The law requires that before a death can be registered for burial or cremation, the medical cause of death must be certified by a doctor who has attended the deceased during the last illness. In most cases, a doctor who was treating the deceased or a general practitioner can issue a medical certificate of the cause of death (MCCD). The death can then be registered under the Births andDeaths Registration Act 1953, and a certificate issued by the registrar for the funeral arrangements.

In cases of sudden deaths, unexplained deaths or deaths occurring in unusual circumstances, a coroner must make an order as to the cause of death before it can be registered for burial or cremation. The coroner decides whether he or she is satisfied with the nature of the death on the basis of the facts already available. If the cause of death cannot still be established, the coroner can arrange for a post mortem and/or arrange to hold an inquest to find the cause of death.

There have been calls for changes to the certification of death and the coronial system. This follows some high-profile cases, such as the conviction of Dr Harold Shipman in 2000 for the murder of many of his patients. One area of concern that has emerged in subsequent inquiries was the lack of safeguards to ensure that suspicious deaths are reported to the coroner and investigated properly. Following the reports of two inquiries, a Coroners and Justice Bill was introduced in December 2008 with the aim of reforming and modernising the coronial system and improving the service.

The aim of this chapter is to understand the issues associated with post mortems and inquests.

LEARNING OUTCOMES

At the end of this chapter, the reader will be able to:

❑ Outline the development of the coronial system.
❑ Outline the main duties of the coroner in relation to reported deaths.
❑ Discuss the process for verifying and certifying death.
❑ Discuss instances when a death should be reported to the coroner.
❑ Discuss the general and statutory duty to report a death to the coroner.
❑ Outline the process by which the coroner establishes the cause of death.
❑ Describe the procedure for a coroner's inquest.
❑ Discuss the background for reform of the coronial system.

DEVELOPMENT OF THE CORONIAL SYSTEM

The office of coroner was formally established in 1194 during the reign of Richard I. The coroner's duty then, apart from investigating sudden deaths, included investigations that could raise revenues for the crown. For example, suicides were investigated, on the grounds that the goods and chattels of those found guilty of the crime of 'self murder' would be forfeited to the crown. Over the centuries, the role of the coroner went through a process of change. Under the Coroners Act of 1887, the role was primarily concerned in determining the circumstances and the medical causes of sudden, violent and unnatural deaths. This role continues today under the Coroners' Rules 1984 and the Coroners Act 1988. Today's coroners enquire and investigate, on behalf of the state, those deaths that are reported to them in order to determine the cause of death.

Coroners are lawyers and some are qualified medical practitioners of no less than five years' experience (section 2 of the Coroners Act 1988). They are appointed and paid by local authorities in each district. Coroners are required to appoint suitably qualified persons to act as their deputies (section 6(1) of the Coroners Act 1988). However, under section 7(1) of the Act, a deputy is only permitted to act for a coroner due to absence from ill-health or any other lawful cause. Suitably qualified persons may also be appointed to act as assistant deputy coroners under section 6(2) of the Act. These assistants are permitted to act in place of the coroner and deputy coroner only when both are absent or where both are unable to act in a particular case.

DUTIES OF A CORONER REGARDING REPORTED DEATHS

The duties of coroners (Box 11.1) are to respond and investigate deaths reported to them. They do not pro-actively screen all deaths and then decide which should be investigated. After a death has been reported, they seek to establish the identity of the deceased, the circumstances surrounding the death and the medical cause of death. A coroner may decide that a reported death is natural and there is a doctor who can sign the medical certificate.

A coroner may also ask for a post mortem to be carried out in order to establish the cause of death. If the result shows that the

---

Box 11.1 Duties of a coroner

- Investigate deaths where the cause is unknown.
- Investigate all deaths where there is reason to believe that the cause of death was violent or unnatural.
- Investigate all deaths that occurred in prison or in such a place or in such circumstances as to require an inquest under any other Act.
- Decide if a post mortem is required and instruct a medical practitioner to undertake it.
- Hold an inquest with or without a jury.
- Inform the registrar of deaths if no inquest is required.
- Inform the registrar of deaths of the result of an inquest.
- Keep a register of all reported deaths and documentation relating to post mortems and inquests.
- Submit an annual report to the Ministry of Justice about deaths investigated, inquests held and any other required information.
- Authorise the exhumation of bodies for criminal investigations.
- Authorise the removal of bodies out of England and Wales.

---

cause of death is due to natural causes, there might not be an inquest and the coroner can complete a form for the death to be registered.

Where the cause of death cannot be established after a post mortem, the coroner will hold an inquest. By law, coroners have a duty to hold an inquest in other circumstances, such as a violent death or death occurring in prison. Other duties of a coroner include the power to authorise the exhumation of bodies in cases of criminal proceedings. If the body of a deceased person needs to be taken out of the country (England and Wales), the coroner must issue an order before the body can be removed.

Coroners are normally responsible for investigating a death only if the body lies within their districts. Whether a coroner becomes involved depends on where the body lies and not where the death occurs. Where a death occurs outside England and Wales, a coroner will become involved if the body is brought into his or her district and where there is reason to suspect that the deceased has died a violent or unnatural death, or has died a sudden death of which the cause is not known.

PROCESS FOR VERIFYING AND CERTIFYING DEATH

Verification of death

Verification of the fact of death is defined as deciding whether a patient is actually deceased. It does not require a medically registered practitioner to undertake this verification. Although a nurse cannot legally certify death, she can confirm that death has occurred. Only experienced registered nurses, with the necessary competencies, skills and knowledge and working within local agreed policies or protocols have the authority to verify the fact of death. The Nursing and Midwifery Council (NMC) (2006) advises that 'a registered nurse may confirm or verify life extinct providing there is an explicit local protocol in place to allow such an action, which includes guidance on when other authorities, e.g. the police or the coroner, should be informed prior to the removal of the body'.

Nurses should only verify death in situations where the death is expected. Expected death is defined as 'death following on from a period of illness which has been identified as terminal, and where no active intervention to prolong life is ongoing' (Ayris, 2002). Those nurses on whom this duty falls should adhere to the NMC code of professional conduct (NMC, 2008). They must also be aware of the legal issues and related account-ability of this extended scope of professional practice.

Certification of death

Certification of death is the process of completing the MCCD, which must be completed by a medical practitioner. The legal position regarding certification of death is determined by the Births and Deaths Registration Act 1953. A registered medical practitioner who has attended a deceased person during his last illness is required to give the MCCD. The doctor does not have to see the body and can ask another professional, such as a nurse, to confirm that death has occurred. The coroner must be informed if a doctor is unwilling or unable to certify the cause of death.

DEATHS THAT SHOULD BE REPORTED TO THE CORONER

Not all deaths are reported to the coroner. In most cases of death, a general practitioner or a hospital doctor can issue the MCCD. Where there is reasonable cause to suspect that the deceased has died a violent or an unnatural death, has died a sudden death of which the cause is unknown, or has died in prison or in such a place or in such circumstances as to require an inquest under any other Act, the coroner should hold an inquest into the death of the deceased (Coroners Act 1988, section 8(1)). Therefore, such deaths must be reported to the coroner so that an inquest can be held.

Prison is not defined and can include other places where the deceased is restrained or deprived of his or her liberty. The Home Office recommends that coroners should hold an inquest into the death of a person in any type of legal custody. The term 'unnatu-ral death' is not defined by statute. In *R v Price* [1884], 'unnatural' was interpreted as 'a reasonable suspicion that there may have been something peculiar about the death; that it may have been due to other causes than common illness'. An example is a death as a result of a drug overdose or suicide.

A death may be considered 'violent' where a person is injured, intentionally or accidentally. This includes deaths due to an accident or where there is reasonable cause to suspect a crime, such as murder. A sudden death with the cause unknown includes an unexpected death where either the terminal cause of death or the underlying medical condition is unknown. Where there is reasonable cause to suspect that a person has died a sudden death, with the cause unknown and the death was not violent, unnatural or occurred in prison, the coroner can order a post mortem. If the post mortem result shows that the death was natural, the coroner does not have to hold an inquest (Coroners Act 1988, section 19(3)). However, there should be an inquest if other statutory requirements to hold an inquest apply.

There are therefore are many situations where, by law, a death must be reported to a coroner for further inquiries into the cause of death. An example is when a patient dies in hospital due to an untoward clinical incident or where a death occurred during an operation or before the patient has recovered from an anaesthetic. Deaths that happen within 24 h of admission to hospital and deaths due to an abortion or a stillbirth (where there was any possibility of the child being born alive) must be reported. Another situation for reporting a death is when no doctor has treated the deceased during his or her last illness. If patients have been treated, the doctor must have seen them within the 14 days before or after the death (28 days in Northern Ireland).

Deaths that may be due to industrial diseases must also be reported to the coroner. An industrial disease is a disease, illness or disability resulting from certain conditions of employment. This is usually due to exposure to physical, biological or chemical agents. Asbestos-related disease is such an example. Deaths due to tetanus, septicaemia or gangrene, where the cause cannot be identified, are also reported, as are deaths due to any kind of poisoning, either deliberate or accidental. Poisoning includes taking an overdose of medicine, ingesting harmful chemicals or inhaling gases, such as carbon monoxide. A death should also be reported where it may be due to the deceased taking illicit drugs, such as those controlled under the Misuse of Drugs Act 1971.

The coroner must be informed where there is suspicion that a death is due to self-neglect or neglect by others. Death due to self-neglect includes instances where vulnerable adults refused help and services despite being at grave risk of harm. Neglect by others, in general, is a gross failure to fulfil one's responsibilities to provide the needed care for someone in a dependent position (*R v North Humberside Coroner ex parte Jamieson* [1995]). This can be active or passive neglect. Active neglect refers to behaviour that is willful, ie the caregiver intentionally withholds care or necessities. Passive neglect refers to situations in which the caregiver is unable to fulfil his or her care-giving responsibilities.

There are situations where there will be uncertainties regarding a decision whether a particular death meets the reporting criteria. There is not a list of all the specific types of death or situations that doctors or nurses could refer to when making such a decision. Whether some deaths should be reported is subject to interpretation because of a lack of clarity in the present legislation. Many coroners issue guidance to medical professionals in their areas, but there is no standard practice. A case that may be referred to a coroner in one area may not necessarily be referred in another area. In practice, this means that coroners have deaths referred to them that should not have been, and deaths which should have been referred are not investigated. The rule of thumb is that if there is any doubt about the cause of death, it should be reported to the coroner. The same rule applies if there are uncertainties about any situations for reporting a death.

DUTY TO REPORT A DEATH TO THE CORONER

To enable coroners to carry out their duties, relevant deaths must be referred to them. Yet there are no direct statutory legal provisions that require any person to report a death to the coroner. Where such statutory duty exists, it is derived from other legislations, such as registration legislation, where the registrar of births and deaths must report certain deaths to the coroner. Other legislations governing prisons impose a duty on a prison governor to inform the coroner of the death of an inmate.

If anyone finds a dead body or is aware that a death was due to unnatural causes or violence, there is a duty to inform the police, who in turn will inform the coroner. The government has produced a consultation paper about the statutory duty for doctors and other public service personnel to report deaths to the coroner. The consultation ended in July 2007.

The majority of cases of deaths are referred to the coroner directly by the police and by doctors. Normally deaths are referred to the coroner where there is reason to suspect that the death was unnatural, violent, sudden with cause unknown, the death relates to the deceased's employment or occurred during or shortly after detention in police or prison custody. Where there are doubts whether a death should be reported, doctors usually report the death and seek the advice of the coroner. Where the coroner has not been informed of a death that should have been reported, the registrar of births, marriages and deaths is under a statutory duty to inform the coroner under registration legislation.

STATUTORY DUTY TO REPORT A DEATH TO THE CORONER

By law, a death must be registered and a certificate issued by the Registrar before the deceased can be buried or cremated (Births and Deaths Registration Act 1953). Registrars of births and deaths are under a legal duty to report certain categories of deaths to the coroner in order for the cause of death to be properly established before they can be registered (Births and Death Regulations 1987, section 41(1)).

To register a death, a duly completed certificate with all the necessary information is required. Where the registrar is unable to obtain a duly completed certificate of the cause of death, the coroner will be informed. A death will also be reported where the deceased was not attended during his or her last illness by a registered medical practitioner or if it appears to the registrar that the deceased was not seen by the doctor who has certified the death either after death or within 14 days before the death. If a death appears to the registrar, from the information given, to be due to an industrial disease or industrial poisoning or it occurred during an operation or before recovery from the effect of an anaesthetic, the coroner will be informed. Where the cause of death appears to be unknown or the registrar has cause to believe that the death is unnatural or has been caused by violence, neglect or the death occurred in suspicious circumstances, it will be reported to the coroner.

ESTABLISHMENT BY THE CORONER OF THE CAUSE OF DEATH

When a death has been reported, the coroner will firstly try to establish that the death was due to natural causes or is satisfied as to the nature of the death. If the coroner chooses not to continue the investigation with an autopsy and/or inquest, he or she informs the registrar and doctor and certification takes place with the coroner's agreement. Once the certificate is issued, the death can be registered and funeral arrangements made.

If the coroner is unable to either establish the cause of death or establish the cause of death as due to natural causes, arrangements will be made for a post-mortem examination (autopsy) to be performed. A post mortem ordered by a coroner must take place by law, whether the next-of-kin gives their agreement or not. The coroner has a duty to notify specified persons or bodies that a post mortem will take place unless it is impracticable to notify any such persons or bodies or to do so would cause the examination to be unduly delayed (Coroners' Rules 1984, Rule 7(1)). These include relatives who have notified the coroner of their wish to attend or be represented, the deceased's general practitioner and the hospital if the death occurred there. If the post-mortem examination shows that the death was due to natural causes, the coroner will certify the death and it can be registered. If the post mortem shows that the death was not due to natural causes or the results are inconclusive, the coroner is obliged to hold an inquest.

PROCEDURE FOR A CORONER'S INQUEST

A coroner's inquest is a legal inquiry into the medical cause and circumstances of a death. During an inquest, the coroner can call upon and examine various witnesses, including doctors, nurses and other healthcare professionals who have relevant information concerning the inquiry. It is held in public unless there is an application for evidence to be heard *in camera*, for example in a case involving the security services.

When required, an inquest must be held in cases where:

- The death was violent or unnatural.
- The death took place in prison or police custody or in circumstances where other statutes require an inquest, such as in criminal cases, in reportable industrial diseases or under health and safety law.
- The cause of death, such as sudden death, is still uncertain after a post mortem.

An inquest is not a trial and the coroner cannot blame anyone for the death. As such, the verdict of an inquest must not apportion criminal or civil liability on someone.

Requirement of a jury

Inquests are generally carried out by the coroner alone although a jury can be called at his or her own discretion. However, under certain circumstances, the coroner is required by law to call a jury (about 7–11 members) for the inquest (section 8(3) of the Coroners Act 1988):

- If the death occurred in prison, in police custody or as a result of an injury caused by a police officer.
- If the death was caused by an accident, poisoning or disease in circumstances which are legally required to be reported to the government (such as a road traffic accident or an industrial accident).
- If the death occurred in circumstances that could have a detrimental effect on the health and safety of the public.

Informing the next of kin

If the coroner decides to have an inquest, he or she must inform amongst others the married or civil partner of the deceased. Otherwise the nearest relative must be informed unless the deceased has no relatives, whereby the personal representative will be informed (Coroners' Rules 1984, Rule 19; Coroners' (Amendment) Rules 2005). Relatives can attend an inquest and ask questions of the witnesses. However, these questions can only be about the medical cause and circumstances of the death. They can also ask a lawyer to represent them, especially in circumstances which could lead to a claim for compensation.

Witnesses at an inquest

It is the duty of the coroner to decide whether to call any witnesses to an inquest. However, anyone who wants to give evidence at an inquest can do so without being summoned. The coroner must be informed beforehand and the evidence to be presented must be relevant to the purpose of the inquest. If the coroner decides that a particular person, such as a nurse, needs to attend the inquest, a request or a formal summon will be sent to that person. A witness who does not attend an inquest could be fined and repeated failure to attend may result in a custodial sentence. Every individual, including nurses, has the right to be represented by their own legal representative at any stage of the proceedings.

Witnesses give evidence under oath and are initially examined by the coroner. A jury can also question a witness. Anyone who has a 'proper interest' (Box 11.2) can also question a witness personally or through a legal representative (Coroners' Rules 1984, Rule 20(1)). However, a Chief Officer of Police may only question a witness through a lawyer. Any question to the witness

---

Box 11.2 Persons who may have a 'proper interest' are:

- A parent, spouse, child, civil partner and anyone acting for the deceased.
- Anyone who will benefit from a life insurance policy of the deceased.
- Any insurer who has issued a life insurance policy.
- Anyone whose actions the coroner believes may have contributed to the death either accidentally or otherwise.
- The Chief of Police.
- Any person appointed by a government department, such as a health and safety inspector.
- A representative of any relevant trade union (if the death arose in connection with the person's employment or was due to industrial disease).
- Anyone else whom the coroner may decide has a 'proper interest'.

---

must be relevant, sensible and should not be accusatory. The questions must relate only to who the deceased was, and how, when and where he or she died. Witnesses can refer to their statements when answering questions and they do not have to answer any question that can incriminate them.

Similarly, where someone is suspected of causing a death and is required to give evidence at an inquest, he or she is protected against answering any question that may incriminate them. The coroner has the final say over what may or may not be asked. Where a witness cannot attend an inquest, a coroner can read to the court the evidence in documentary form as long as the evidence is unlikely to be disputed and there is no objection from any interested party.

Coroner's verdict following an inquest

Following inquests, coroners record their or the jury's verdict as to how the deceased came to his or her death. The coroner or jury certifies the facts of the death on an inquisition form. It is not a verdict about whether someone is guilty of an offence because the coroner is restricted from framing a verdict in such a way, which would appear to attribute either civil liability or criminal liability on the part of a named person. The coroner's inquest is inquisitorial and the coroner's duty is to enquire as to the cause of the death and the circumstances in which it occurred. The following are examples of the types of verdict that coroners might return following an inquest:

- *Death by misadventure:* a death that is unintentional, resulting from an intentional and lawful action, e.g. medical intervention.
- *Accidental death:* a death resulting from an accident where neither the action nor the death was intended.
- *Unlawful killing:* a death caused by another person, without lawful excuse and in breach of the criminal law, such as murder, manslaughter, gross negligence.
- *Lawful killing:* a death due to lawful justification, such as in self-defence.
- *Death by natural causes:* a death caused by a naturally occurring disease or illness.

- *Suicide:* a death due to an intentional act of terminating one's own life. If at the time of the death the deceased was suffering from a psychiatric condition, the coroner may record that the deceased killed himself or herself whilst the balance of the deceased's mind was disturbed.
- *Open verdict:* a verdict where there is insufficient evidence for any other verdict.
- *Attempted/self-induced abortion:* a death resulting from a self-induced unlawful abortion.
- *Still birth:* a verdict given in the case of a baby who has not breathed or shown any actual signs of life after delivery (after 24 weeks).
- *Want of attention at birth:* a death resulting from lack of attention at birth. An example will be when a baby died when the mother gave birth alone without any medical supervision.
- *Narrative verdict:* when the coroner is unsure as to what caused the death. The coroner records the circumstances surrounding the death.
- *Neglect verdict:* a death due to gross failure to provide adequate care to someone requiring that care. This verdict can only be added to another one, such as 'death by misadventure due to neglect'.

Actions following a verdict

There is no criminal or civil liability following the verdict of a coronial inquest. Sometimes the inquest will show that something needs to be done to prevent a recurrence of fatalities. Under Rule 43 of the Coroners' Rules 1984, a coroner may announce at the inquest that he or she is reporting to a person or authority any actions that the coroner believes should be taken to prevent a recurrence of fatalities that have been enquired at the inquest. This is done to prevent more deaths under similar circumstances. The coroner can draw attention to these publicly and to any appropriate person or authority, such as an NHS Trust or to an inspector appointed under section 19 of the Health and Safety at Work Act 1974.

Under the provisions of the Coroners' (Amendment) Rules 2008, a new statutory duty has been placed on organisations to respond to a coroner's concerns within 56 days. Coroners must share reports and responses with those, including bereaved families, to whom they have assigned interested person status. Reports and information can also be shared with the Lord Chancellor and other interested organisations. These reports and responses will be centrally collated so that the lessons learned can be disseminated widely.

The 2008 rules also require coroners to notify Local Safeguarding Children Boards of any child death that is reported to them and to share information, such as reports from post-mortem examinations and documents given in evidence at an inquest, with these child protection bodies. This will enable Local Safeguarding Children Boards to meet their statutory duty to conduct child death reviews and to implement the lessons learned from inquests concerning the death of a child more widely.

There is no right of appeal from a coroner's decision except by way of a judicial review. For example in *Sacker v HM Coroner for West Yorkshire* [2003], Mrs Helen Sacker, the mother of a prisoner who had committed suicide, sought a judicial review of the coroner's decision not to return a verdict of neglect. The inquest decision was quashed and a fresh inquest ordered.

BACKGROUND FOR REFORM OF THE CORONIAL SYSTEM

There has been public concern about the effectiveness of the coronial system, especially following the conviction of Dr Harold Shipman in 2000. Many of his patients died suddenly in circumstances where the deaths should have been investigated. He was able to certify the cause of death and avoid any official enquiry into the deaths. An inquiry was set up in February 2001 under the chairmanship of Dame Janet Smith to establish what changes need to be put in place to protect patients in the future. Part of the inquiry was to examine the works of the coroners and the death certification system. Another review under the chairmanship of Tom Luce, focusing on death certification and coroner services, was also set up in July 2001.

The *Fundamental Review of Death Certification and Investigation* (Home Office, 2003) and the *Third Report of the Shipman Inquiry* (The Shipman Inquiry, 2003) identified a number of issues with the present service, which need reform. According to the reports, the present system lacks leadership, safeguards and quality control. Families are often excluded in coroners' investigations and there is a lack of medical support for coroners. Moreover in the present system, death certification and investigation are separate from each other. There is no means of ensuring that a death that ought to be reported to a coroner for investigation is so reported. A coroner has no jurisdiction to investigate deaths not reported to him or her. There are therefore inadequate safeguards against a doctor 'certifying his way out of trouble'.

In 2004, the government drew on recommendations from both reports to produce a position paper 'Reforming the coroner and death certification service'. The Department for Constitutional Affairs announced in June 2006 its intention to proceed with the reform of the coronial system and published a draft Coroners' Bill. After extensive consultation, a number of policy areas in the Bill were revised and a new Coroners and Justice Bill was introduced in December 2008.

Some of the main recommendations of the two reports were not included in the Bill. The government has not reformed the system of death certification in the way recommended by the reviews. The Bill instead includes some measures to simplify death certification by making the process more transparent. Other reforms include the improvement of the service provided to the bereaved, a national framework and leadership to oversee the system, and more effective investigations and inquests.

Coroners and Justice Bill – some key reforms
Charters
To improve the coronial service, a coroners' charter will set out guidelines and standards about the service bereaved people can expect. It will also promote better contact between them and the service. The rights of the bereaved in relation to coronial investigations and what they can expect from the system will be set out in a charter (Bereaved People Charter). The service aims to be sensitive to the needs of the bereaved family. For example, to avoid increasing the grief of bereaved people in cases of suicides or child death cases, the current code of conduct by the media will be refined to ensure that there is appropriate emphasis on sensitive reporting. Families can complain if they feel any provisions in the code have been breached.

Rights of bereaved people and the coroners' investigations
One of the key reforms in the Bill is to enable relatives of the deceased to contribute to coroners' investigations to a greater extent. They will have new rights to appeal against matters and decisions that concern them. The Bill creates a new appeals system and provides a new simple route for bereaved people to challenge coroners' decisions.

Coronial staff
A new chief coroner, accountable to the government, will be appointed to lead the coronial service on a national basis. The duties of the chief coroner will include the consideration of appeals against coroners' decisions, responding to complaints and supporting local coroners. The chief coroner will also be responsible for developing national standards and guidance in order for the service to function effectively and to advise the government on issues relating to the service.

The hierarchy under the 1988 Act of coroners, deputy coroners and assistant deputy coroners will change to senior coroners, area coroners and assistant coroners. All coroners must be legally qualified and will become full-time. The current boundaries of the coroner will be reshaped to ensure effective operation and coordination with other statutory services, such as the police. A 'coroner for treasure' for England and Wales will be appointed. The aim of this is to release local coroner resources to focus on the investigation of deaths.

Coronial Advisory Council
A new council, to be known as the Coronial Advisory Council, will provide advice and make recommendations to the chief coroner and Lord Chancellor on policy and operational matters relating to the coroners' service. It is intended that this council will include members of the public who have had dealings with the service.

Circumstances to investigate death
Although the circumstances in which a coroner must investigate a death are broadly similar to those in section 8(1) of the Coroners Act 1988, there are some changes in the Bill. The requirement

under section 8(1) (b) of the Act that a death be 'sudden', as well as of a 'cause unknown', has been removed. There will therefore be a duty to investigate both expected and sudden deaths if the coroner has reasonable cause to suspect that the cause of death is unknown.

The requirement to investigate a death that has occurred in prison under section 8(1) (c) of the Act has also been changed so that it will apply to deaths where the deceased was in prison or otherwise detained in custody. Detention in custody will include detention in a police cell, immigration detention centre and detention under mental health legislation.

Duty to hold an investigation and an inquest
The coroner's duty to hold an investigation and the duty to hold an inquest will be separated. The Bill permits the coroner to open an investigation, but not to proceed to a full-scale inquest where the coroner does not consider that such an inquiry is justifiable. The relatives of the deceased may, however, challenge that decision by way of appeal.

Post mortem
There are new powers in respect of post-mortem examinations. The coroner can arrange to move bodies to any place for a post mortem rather than as at present just within his or her area or a neighbouring area. This is aimed at enabling coroners to make better use of specialist pathology skills and specialist equipment where an investigation into a particular death requires it.

The Bill also does away with the distinction between post-mortem and 'special' examinations. Coroners will be able to be more specific about the kind of examination they would like doctors to make, such as a particular examination of a tissue or organ if this seems relevant to the cause of death.

Appeal against a coroner's decision
Under the current system there are no means to appeal a coroner's decision or judgement, except for a judicial review. In the Bill, a wide class of 'interested persons', including, but not limited to, the bereaved, will have a right to appeal to the chief coroner about the outcome of an inquest or a decision made by a coroner

in connection with an investigation. For example, a decision not to hold a post mortem will be subject to appeal. The chief coroner will also have powers to compel the coroner to hold an inquest or to quash a verdict from a previous inquest.

Powers to obtain information

During the course of an investigation, coroners will have new powers to obtain information to assist their investigations. There are provisions for coroners to have increased powers to require information to be provided to them and new powers to enter and search premises, and seize property. However, the coroner will have to obtain authorisation from the chief coroner in order to exercise these powers.

Juries

The Bill reduces the numbers of jurors required for a coroner's jury. There must be no fewer than seven and no more than nine jurors. A jury must be summoned where the deceased died while in custody or as a result of an act or omission of a police officer in the purported execution of his or her duty or of a service police officer in the purported execution of his or her duty. An inquest may also be held with a jury in other circumstances where the senior coroner thinks there is sufficient reason for doing so.

Witnesses

Coroners will also be able to take evidence from someone under 17 years of age via live links in a courtroom cleared of everyone except interested persons and the jury. Witnesses over the age of 17 years may also be allowed by the coroner to give evidence through live links, but only if the coroner is satisfied that it would contribute to the efficient administration of the proceedings at the inquest. The evidence from a witness given by live link should be given the same weight as if given at the inquest.

Witnesses must normally give evidence on oath although children under 14 years do not have to give evidence on oath. If the coroner thinks that someone does not have sufficient understanding of the responsibility to tell the truth, they do not have to give evidence on oath.

Certifying death

The overall process for certifying deaths will include guidance that will clarify the criteria for reporting a death to the coroner. This will reduce the number of different criteria being used when deciding whether or not a death should be reported to the coroner. There will be greater availability of coroners to deal with inquiries. Medical advice and expertise will also be more readily available to coroners and will include a chief medical adviser for the coronial service.

Exhumation of a body for examination

Coroners currently have the power to order the exhumation of buried human remains (section 23 of the 1988 Act) for criminal proceedings. In the Bill, coroners will also have the power to allow exhumation for the purposes of investigating the death of someone other than the deceased whose body is to be exhumed.

CONCLUSION

The duties of coroners are to enquire and investigate, on behalf of the state, those deaths reported to them in order to determine the cause of death. Experienced and competent registered nurses, working within local agreed policies or protocols can verify the fact of death. Only a doctor can certify death. By law, a violent or unnatural death, a sudden death with the cause unknown and death in prison must be reported to the coroner. When a death is reported, a coroner will firstly try to establish if the death was due to natural causes. If not, the coroner can order a post mortem to establish the cause of death.

A coroner's inquest is a legal inquiry into the medical cause and circumstances of a death. Inquests can be held with or without a jury but under certain circumstances the coroner is required by law to call a jury.

Following inquests, coroners record their or the jury's verdict as to how the deceased came to his or her death. No civil or criminal liability is attributed to a named person. A coroner may inform a person or authority of any actions that the coroner believes should be taken to prevent a recurrence of fatalities.

Concerns about the effectiveness of the coronial system and subsequent reports of two reviews led to the production of the Coroners and Justice Bill 2008.

The aims of the Bill are to modernise the coronial service. It includes some reforms, such as improving the service provided to the bereaved, a national framework and leadership to oversee the coronial system, and more effective investigations and inquests about the cause of death.

REFERENCES

Ayris W (2002) Verification of expected death by district nurses. *Br J Community Nurs* **7**(7): 370–373.

Coroners' Rules 1984 (SI 1984/552).

Coroners' (Amendment) Rules 2005 (SI 2005/420).

Coroners (Amendment) Rules 2008 (SI 2008/1652).

Department for Constitutional Affairs (2006) *Coroner Reform: The Government's Draft Bill: Improving death investigation in England and Wales, Cm 6849*. The Stationery Office, London.

Home Office (2003) *Death Certification and Investigation in England, Wales and Northern Ireland The Report of a Fundamental Review (Cmd 5831)*. The Stationery Office, London.

Nursing and Midwifery Council (NMC) (2006) *Advice Sheet on Death Certification*. NMC, London.

Nursing and Midwifery Council (NMC) (2008) *The Code: Standards of conduct, performance and ethics for nurses and midwives*. NMC, London.

R v Coroner for North Humberside and Scunthorpe ex parte Jamieson [1995] QB1y.

R v Price (1884) 12 QBD 247.

Registration of Births and Death Regulations (1987) (SI 1987/2088).

Sacker v Her Majesty's Coroner for the County of West Yorkshire [2003] Lloyd's Rep Med 326.

The Shipman Inquiry (2003) *Third Report Death Certification and the Investigation of Deaths by Coroners, Cm 5854*. The Stationery Office, London.

Record Keeping* | **12**

Philip Jevon

INTRODUCTION

'Record keeping is an integral part of nursing, midwifery and health visiting practice. It is a tool of professional practice and one that should help the care process. It is not separate from this process and it is not an optional extra to be fitted in if circumstances allow.'

(Nursing and Midwifery Council (NMC), 2005)

Accurate record keeping is paramount when caring for a dying patient and when encountering a death, e.g. what has been communicated to the patient and next of kin concerning prognosis, the issuing of a 'do not attempt resuscitation' order, time of death, who was present at the death, who certified the patient, what jewellery was left on the body prior to transfer to the mortuary, etc., must be correctly and accurately documented. The nurse must ensure that accurate and good records are kept.

The aim of this chapter is to understand good record keeping.

LEARNING OUTCOMES

At the end of the chapter, the reader will be able to:

❑ Discuss the importance of good record keeping.
❑ List the common deficiencies in record keeping.
❑ Discuss the principles of good record keeping.
❑ Outline the legal issues associated with record keeping.
❑ Outline the NMC statement on record keeping.

*This chapter is based on the chapter 'Record Keeping', which first appeared in *Monitoring the Critically Ill Patient* by Jevon & Ewens (2007).

IMPORTANCE OF GOOD RECORD KEEPING

Good record keeping will help to protect the welfare of both the patient and the nurse by promoting:

- High standards of clinical care.
- Continuity of care.
- Better communication and dissemination of information between members of the interprofessional healthcare team.
- The ability to detect problems, such as changes in the patient's condition, at an early stage.
- An accurate account of treatment and care planning and delivery.

The quality of record keeping is also a reflection on the standard of nursing practice: good record keeping is an indication that the practitioner is professional and skilled, while poor record keeping often highlights wider problems with the individual's practice (NMC, 2005).

COMMON DEFICIENCIES IN RECORD KEEPING

Nearly every report published by the Health Service Commissioner (Health Service Ombudsman) following a complaint identifies examples of poor record keeping that has either hampered the care the patient has received or has made it difficult for healthcare professionals to defend their practice (Dimond, 2005).

Common deficiencies in record keeping encountered include:

- Absence of clarity.
- Failure to record action taken when a problem has been identified.
- Missing information.
- Spelling mistakes.
- Inaccurate records.

(Dimond, 2005)

PRINCIPLES OF GOOD RECORD KEEPING

There are a number of factors that underpin good record keeping. The patient's records should:

- Be factual, consistent and accurate.
- Be updated as soon as possible after any recordable event.

- Provide current information on the care and condition of the patient.
- Be documented clearly and in such a way that the text cannot be erased.
- Be consecutive and accurately dated, timed and signed (including a printed signature).
- Have any alterations and additions dated, timed and signed; all original entries should be clearly legible.
- Not include abbreviations, jargon, meaningless phrases, irrelevant speculation and offensive subjective statements.
- Still be legible if photocopied.
- Identify any problems identified and most importantly the action taken to rectify them.

Best practice – record keeping
Records must be:

- Factual.
- Legible.
- Clear.
- Concise.
- Accurate.
- Signed.
- Timed.
- Dated.

(Drew *et al.*, 2000)

LEGAL ISSUES ASSOCIATED WITH RECORD KEEPING
The patient's records are occasionally required as evidence before a court of law, by the Health Service Commissioner or in order to investigate a complaint at a local level. Sometimes they may be requested by the NMC's Fitness to Practice committees when investigating complaints related to misconduct. Care plans, diaries and anything that makes reference to the patient's care may be required as evidence (NMC, 2005).

What constitutes a legal document is often a cause for concern. Any document requested by the court becomes a legal document (Dimond, 1994), e.g. nursing records, medical records, X-rays, laboratory reports, observation charts; in fact any document that may be relevant to the case.

If any of the documents are missing, the writer of the records may be cross-examined as to the circumstances of their disappearance (Dimond, 1994). 'Medical records are not proof of the truth of the facts stated in them but the maker of the records may be called to give evidence as to the truth as to what is contained in them' (Dimond, 1994).

The approach to record keeping adopted by courts of law tends to be that if it is not recorded, it has not been undertaken (NMC, 2005). Professional judgement is required when deciding what is relevant and what needs to be recorded, particularly if the patient's clinical condition is apparently unchanging and no record has been made of the care that has been delivered.

A registered nurse has both a professional and a legal duty of care. Consequently, when keeping records it is important to be able to demonstrate that:

- A comprehensive nursing assessment of the patient has been undertaken, including care that has been planned and provided.
- Relevant information is included, together with any measures that have been taken in response to changes in the patient's condition.
- The duty of care owed to the patient has been honoured and that no acts or omissions have compromised the patient's safety.
- Arrangements have been made for ongoing care of the patient.

The registered nurse is also accountable for any delegation of record keeping to members of the multiprofessional team who are not registered practitioners. For example, if record keeping is delegated to a pre-registration student nurse or a healthcare assistant, competence to perform the task must be ensured and adequate supervision provided. All such entries must be countersigned.

The Access to Health Records Act 1990 gives patients the right of access to their manually maintained health records which were made after 1 November 1991. The Data Protection Act 1998 gives patients the right to access their computer-held records. The

Freedom of Information Act 2000 grants the rights to anyone to all information that is not covered by the Data Protection Act 1998 (NMC, 2005).

Sometimes it is necessary to withhold information if it could affect the physical or mental well-being of the patient or if it would breach another patient's confidentiality (NMC, 2005). If the decision to withhold information is made, justification for doing so must be clearly recorded in the patient's notes.

NMC STATEMENT ON RECORD KEEPING

In *The Code, Standards Of Conduct, Performance And Ethics For Nurses And Midwives* (NMC, 2008), it states that all nurses and midwives must:

- Keep clear and accurate records.
- Keep clear and accurate records of the discussions they have, the assessments they make, the treatment and medicines they give and how effective these have been.
- Complete records as soon as possible after an event has occurred.
- Not tamper with original records in any way.
- Ensure any entries they make in an individual's paper records are clearly and legibly signed, dated and timed.
- Ensure any entries they make in an individual's electronic records are clearly attributable to them.
- Ensure all records are kept confidentially and securely.

CONCLUSION

This chapter has provided an overview to good record keeping. The importance of good record keeping has been discussed. The common deficiencies in record keeping have been highlighted and the principles of good record keeping have been discussed. The legal issues associated with record keeping have been outlined.

REFERENCES

Dimond B (1994) *Legal Aspects in Midwifery*. Midwifery Press, Cheshire.
Dimond B (2005) Exploring common deficiencies that occur in record keeping. *Br J Nurs* **14**(10): 568–570.

Drew D, Jevon P, Raby M (2000) *Resuscitation of the Newborn*. Butterworth Heinemann, Oxford.

Jevon P, Ewens B (2007) *Monitoring the Critically Ill Patient*. 2nd edn. Blackwell Publishing, Oxford.

Nursing and Midwifery Council (NMC) (2005) *Guidelines for Records and Record Keeping*. NMC, London.

Nursing and Midwifery Council (NMC) (2008) *The Code, Standards of Conduct, Performance and Ethics for Nurses and Midwives*. NMC, London.

Index